Praise for *How to Prepare for Home Birth*

○ ○ ○ ○ ○ ○ ○ ○ ● ● ● ● ● ● ○ ○ (○

"In each of these beautiful birth stories there is a common thread of courage, strength, and trust in the magnificence of the work that is childbirth. We are not broken, we are strong, we are powerful, and we can move mountains when we get to birth on our terms."

—Tracy Donegan, midwife and founder of GentleBirth

"Reading this so-needed collection of very real but inspiring and deeply positive home birth stories was like reading about the births I have attended over the decades in my midwifery practice. I could picture each one as if I was there. There was love, laughter, tears, and such joy and gratitude—and my heart smiled. What a wonderful way to spread awareness, dispel myths, and alleviate common fears about home birth with well-trained and experienced midwives! There are stories for just about everyone: first timers; experienced moms opting for a better experience than previous ones in hospital; moms who had prior cesarean births; single, same sex, young, and older moms; moms with a variety of complications or variations of normal; moms with hard births; moms with easy gentle births; and a variety of dads. But there are common threads that can reassure, encourage, and even excite home birth families; words like calm, peaceful, beautiful, magical, ecstatic, empowering, transformative, exhilarating; as well as phrases like 'It was the most spectacular moment of my life' and 'I would do it again without hesitation.' Women felt incredibly safe, confident in the process, and supported like goddesses. They found their inner warrior strength and capabilities, and loved their experiences despite the challenges. What a powerful resource for those who are considering or planning home birth!"

—Anne Margolis, certified nurse midwife,
founder of HomeSweetHomebirth.com

"For those who never tire of reading a good birth story, this book is for you. It also is for women who are considering a home birth and want to hear about what to expect and how the experience has the potential to transform their lives."

—Cheryl K. Smith, managing editor of *Midwifery Today*

"*How to Prepare for Home Birth* is in a class all its own. Families who choose home birth do so for a myriad of reasons. This book tells the tales while being honest, candid, and sometimes hilarious. Labor is always different, no two people are alike, and birth communities vary from place to place. This book will help bring understanding to anyone looking to find out just how different home birth families can be, from maverick to medical. I give this book two thumbs up!"

—Jessica Thompson, president and
cofounder of SaferBirthinBama.org

"A wonderful compilation of home birth stories from the United States and Europe. The stories discuss why women choose home birth, their struggles to find a midwife, and even their fears. It is a realistic collection of stories that will inspire you to see home birth as normal."

—W. Yvonne Silbernagel, certified professional midwife

HOW TO PREPARE FOR
HOME
BIRTH

*The Joy of Having Babies
at Home for Health and
Well-Being*

SHANTEL SILBERNAGEL

Skyhorse Publishing

Skyhorse Publishing books may be purchased in bulk at special discounts for sales promotion, corporate gifts, fund-raising, or educational purposes. Special editions can also be created to specifications. For details, contact the Special Sales Department, Skyhorse Publishing, 307 West 36th Street, 11th Floor, New York, NY 10018 or info@skyhorsepublishing.com.

Skyhorse® and Skyhorse Publishing® are registered trademarks of Skyhorse Publishing, Inc.®, a Delaware corporation.

Visit our website at www.skyhorsepublishing.com.

10 9 8 7 6 5 4 3 2 1

Library of Congress Cataloging-in-Publication Data is available on file.

Cover design by Daniel Brount

Cover photos by Ryan Silbernagel, Pip Bacon of Purple Raspberry Photography, Patricia Madden, Justin Acharya, Shalome Stone, Rekita Bradley, Bobbie Grove, Samyra P., Chastidy Berg, Becky Clissmann, Karyn Loftesness Photography, Lyn Estall, Neil Dunne, Jessica, Karen Thurston, Stunt Double Creative, Karen Wulf, Laura Nichols LM CPM, Rebekah Lehman of Kindred Photo & Design, Jen Marlow LM CPM, Vania Stoyanova, Vania Photo Studio, Milli Hill, Tracy Lyons, Bronwen Howley Photography, Dembinska-Lemus, Laura Armstrong Photography, and Christy-Joy Ras

Print ISBN: 978-1-5107-5143-9
Ebook ISBN: 978-1-5107-5145-3

Printed in the United States of America

This book is dedicated to nature and all it has to teach us.
Also, to my parents, my husband, and our children; your support is everything.

Contents

○ ○ ○ ○ ○ ○ ○ ○ ○ ○ ○ ○ ○ ○ ○ ○ ○ ○ ○

Introduction

○ ○ ○ ○ ○ ○ ○ ○ ○ ○ ○ ○ ○ ○ ○ ○ ○ ○

My dream of assembling and publishing a collection of positive home birth stories began six years ago, when my husband and I decided to have a home birth with our first child and my parents' first grandchild. I'm not sure which produced more fear: our impending birth, or telling my mom about our choice to have a home birth. Interestingly, many of the women I interviewed for this book recounted a similar moment of fear when deciding to tell their mothers about choosing home birth. Not surprisingly, most mothers responded with admiration for their daughters, and the choice of having a home birth opened a dialogue about birth that hadn't existed before. That is truly the beauty of this project. Although the main goal of this collection is to showcase the many women around the world choosing home birth and to provide positive home birth stories for those embarking or considering to embark on a home birth, it has also grown into a grassroots movement that engages women in honest and open discussions about home birth and its transformative power.

This book will not present statistics or other scientific measures regarding the benefits of birthing at home. There are several books, studies, and articles that can provide that important information. This book will provide you with what is lacking in the home birth community: a collection of positive home birth stories to inspire, encourage, and support you and your choice to have a home birth regardless of location, race, socioeconomic status, religion, or marital status. My greatest hope is that you read each home birth story, laugh, cry, feel inspired, keep it on your nightstand to re-read until you welcome your new baby into your home, and then promptly share the book with the first pregnant lady you see walking down the street!

I mentioned that my husband and I decided to have our first baby at home. I was twenty-five years old at the time. It was my first year as a high school English teacher, and we were in the middle of remodeling our little home. In addition to our busy life, our daughter came four weeks early. She was delivered without complications or fear. After telling my mom about our choice to have a home birth, my fear of the actual birth disappeared. We were secure in our choice, had complete confidence in our experienced midwives, and felt in control of the birth. My only wish is that I could have read positive home birth stories that were contemporary and reflective of a wide range of women and situations. As an avid reader and lover of literature, I know the power of a good story. Many read to educate themselves, to vicariously explore foreign ideas, and to be inspired. Even after my own three beautiful home births, and reading hundreds of home birth stories, I continue to be inspired and moved when a mom recounts her journey through labor and birth. Each story is unique, yet strong themes run through them all: a deep understanding that their bodies were made to birth their babies, that experienced and educated midwives bring peace with their mere presence, and that home birth is transformative.

All my best,
Shantel

Why?

A Poem

By Jenny McKinney Philpott, photographer,
HypnoBirthing practitioner, and yoga teacher

I can't understand,
If it is so full of pain,
I can't understand,
What there is to gain?

Why do you want,
To do it again?
How do you know,
If it will be the same?

I don't, I sigh.
But I can try.
Why do I love to carry and birth?
This is why.

It is what I do,
What I am for.
I have no sport, that I adore.

But this, this pushes me,
To the absolute end.
Between here and there,
I completely transcend.

How does it start? You ask.
I really don't know.
Is it me?
Is it baby?
Who decides to go?

Do we need to direct?
Do we need to know?
Do we need to be impatient,
When things go slow?

Erratic. Stopping. Starting.
Overdue. Don't get me wrong,
It's hard, it's tiring,
And it can be long.
But this isn't an equation.

Due date?
This is Mother Nature;
She's allowed to be late.

And when she arrives,
She is like a storm.
Tropical,
Strong, and warm.

And then a blizzard that leaves me,
Silenced with pain.
But still,
I can breathe through the rain.

Because this is what I am for.
I don't play on a team.
I'm better alone.
I need the space to listen to the tone,

Of silence.

I'm in my ruck,
On the ground.
But there's no one on top,
I don't make a sound.

Breathe.

I see the beach. The waves.
The universe. The stars.
How long am I there? I don't know.
Minutes. Hours.

And then, it's time.

This is it.
I have trained nine long months for this event.
Every sickly morning, every book I've read,
Every kick in my belly,
To remind me of the gift I've been sent.

There's a pause,
Relief.
Move, move, move! As I know this pause,
Will be all too brief.

I step into the ring,
But it has no ropes, no bell, no round.
This ring is full of water,
In which I will make my sound.

I change. I morph,
Back to a mammal.
Cataclysmic energy,
I start to channel.

Breathe.

Like every female,
That has gone before.
In this moment, we are together bound.
Then I begin to roar.

Because I am the lion,
The king of the pack.
I am a goddess,
Just sit back.

This is my time,
To reach the Earth's core.
As the energy builds,
More and more.

Leave me, watch me,
Bring life to this earth
This is how,
I was made to birth

And there she is,
A beautiful girl.
I come back to Earth,
After this whirl.

This is my sport. I train. I go head-to-head.
She is my trophy, my first-place golden cup.
I never gave up. I pushed on.
And like a winning athlete, I lift her up.

I step from the ring,
Battered, bloody, but not beat.
I've taken on the universe,
And won. Now, men, that's to be admired.

And every birth is a win.
So for all of my sisters who have brought new life,
Whether you are young, old,
Girlfriend, or wife
I salute you!

Chapter 1

First-Time Mamas Choose Home Birth

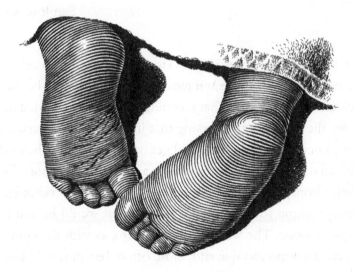

Lucia's Birth

o o o o o o O o o o o o o o o O o

"We are all different, and every birth is unique regardless of location. It's so important to feel like you have a team of women who've gone before you, cheering you on!"
—Amanda, Lucia and Sierra's mama
San Jose, California

Our story begins on Saturday, April 11th. I was forty-one weeks and one day pregnant and feeling more and more like each day could be the day my body decided to get to work. That morning, Brian and I decided to get out of town for the day, secretly thinking that if we distanced ourselves from home a bit, Lucia might take note and get on the move. We headed out to Pescadero, an adorable coastal town with a great country store for lunch, lots of little shops, and the ocean breeze. The drive was calming, and allowed Brian and me some time to relish in what would be some of our final moments alone. The weather in Pescadero, as with the entire Pacific coastline, can be unpredictable and, more often than not, cold and fogged in. That day was perfection! The weather was in the mid-60s and sunny with clear blue skies. We enjoyed lunch, walked around to all the shops, and enjoyed a few moments at the beach with the ocean air in our faces and waves crashing—it was the perfect afternoon.

It was on our drive home that I began feeling some very subtle cramps. I'd had similar cramps on a few separate occasions in the weeks prior; they had lasted a few hours and then tapered off. As the cramps became more consistent, I made a note of the dashboard time and began to notice a pattern of about twenty minutes apart, lasting only ten to fifteen seconds. I was almost positive these would taper off as the others had. Sure enough, by 10:00 p.m. they had passed. We went to bed as usual.

Sunday morning rolled around and Brian and I enjoyed some kitty snuggles while having our weekly phone check-in with his parents. We made a plan to get out of the house again for the afternoon; we decided to go bowling and then to brunch. It was over my bowl of cereal that I started to feel the same kind of cramps I'd felt the day before, but these were inconsistent in both length and duration.

I remembered our doula saying many times, "Don't pay attention to your labor until you have too."

So, that's what I did.

I told Brian I was having cramps again but that we should proceed with our plans. Off we went to the bowling alley! At about 10:00 a.m. and halfway through our second game, I began to track the contractions. Yes, I had officially transitioned from calling them cramps to contractions. I was on board with the idea that this could be the start of early labor. I grabbed my phone, downloaded the first contraction tracker app I found, and continued playing. By the end of our third game, a pattern had emerged: four to five minutes apart and lasting about thirty to forty seconds. This was certainly early labor, but manageable, as I was still playing and talking during contractions. We finished up our fourth game, talked about what we wanted to do, and decided it was going to be a long day/night: best to fuel up with a good meal and enjoy brunch!

By the end of our meal, it was just after 1:00 p.m. and the contractions had intensified a little, making it no longer pleasant to be away from home. Once back at our house, Brian made a to-do list, I made a short grocery list, and then I called our midwife and doula to let them know things were moving. Our doula let us know she was on her way home and that she'd be on standby for us. At this point, I was still in control with contractions being five to six minutes apart and lasting thirty to forty-five seconds; however, I needed to stop and lean on something while I rode each wave. I got Brian out the door to the market for the few things we needed.

I remember telling Brian, "get in, get out, get back, I'm gonna need you!"

I vacuumed the house and sat on my birthing ball at my computer for a little while. Once Brian was back, he sat with me and sent some work emails; it was clear he would not be going in to the office Monday morning.

Around 4:30 p.m. we decided to go for a short walk around the block to get some air. We stopped for the occasional contraction. Leaning on Brain's shoulders and swaying as he hummed to my breathing was a huge relief; it was like dancing in the street! It's one of my favorite memories of that day.

It was after 5:00 p.m. when we got home. I hadn't been timing the contractions for a while, so I decided to move into our bedroom and put on some music to see how far apart they were; four minutes apart, lasting forty-five to fifty seconds, with more intensity that required more focus on my breathing and more aggressive swaying during each contraction. In anticipation of a long night ahead, I hesitantly tried to lie down for a nap. Meanwhile, Brian got to work setting up the birthing tub.

Lying down stunk! I stayed for three contractions and abandoned ship on resting. Convinced I was still in control, I ventured out of our room to ask Brian something between contractions and got caught in the hallway by a big one. I put my hands to the wall and leaned over swaying my hips and trying to remember to breath.

Once it had passed I told Brian, "Okay, that one was bad. I'm officially coping well, but only if I stay really focused between them. I'm going back to the bedroom. You should call our doula."

I shut myself up in our bedroom with my birth playlist (mostly Kirtan music and mantra chants) and a stack of pillows at the end of our bed. I leaned over the pillows on my forearms and just kept breathing and swaying. When our doula arrived, I was still coping well, now on my knees leaned over the glider ottoman from the nursery, rocking back-and-forth with each wave of sensation as Brian put pressure on my hips. I was drifting into labor land, the rest of the world getting very hazy. I soon needed to vocalize through contractions; our doula helped remind me to keep the sound low and to breathe down. The pressure in my bum was increasing, I could tell the desire to push was coming, but didn't know what that meant or if I even should. In the months leading up to our birth, I had immersed myself in education about the stages of labor, the signs for each, average duration, stations of the baby, and dilation, but in the moment, I couldn't tell where I was. I could only feel what my body was driving me to do. Move this way, that way, pressure here, break, drink, move again.

I felt torn between thinking *wow, this is moving much faster than I expected* and *this is only the beginning; stay focused, it's a long road ahead.*

I couldn't decide which thought to believe. I was in the zone, but silently craving guidance. A while later, I had to use the toilet. Taking advantage of the precious time between contractions, we moved in that direction.

I lost my mucus plug just as we got into the bathroom, and I thought to myself, *well, that's progress!*

I had three or four contractions while there, and they were intense. My fuzzy memory still registers those as the worst contractions of the entire experience. I hung onto our doula's waist with all I had while Brian actively filled the birth tub. It was just after 7:00 p.m. now, and our midwife was on her way!

In the break of contractions, I attempted to move to the tub we set up in the nursery. I got as far as the hallway, maybe five steps, before another wave took me to my hands and knees. The contraction passed, and I practically leaped into the tub just a few steps away. Just like all position changes, the initial shock of getting in the tub was uncomfortable! A contraction hit right as I was kneeling down, causing me to lung toward the edge of the tub and grab hold of Brian. Once in a comfortable position, the relief of the water surrounded me, and I was able to refocus. I gripped the back of Brian's arm and the side of the tub as each contraction washed over me; I was breathing and moaning and had genuinely begun to push. The pressure in my bum was incredibly intense, and I was mentally struggling to understand where I was in the process. I remember after a particularly difficult contraction, hearing our midwife's voice for the first time. She was guiding me to bring my tone down, to breathe down, that baby was making her way out, and baby would be here soon.

The recognition of her voice brought me out of my headspace for a moment and I said, "Really, does that mean I'm fully dilated?"

To my recollection, our midwife's response was, "Oh, honey, yes! I couldn't find your cervix if I wanted to. You can check for yourself, baby's head is really close."

Upon personal investigation, she was one hundred percent correct. Our baby's head was very close. With that knowledge, I suddenly knew that all the pressure I was feeling was really my baby's head! That knowledge was empowering! With each contraction, I was able to push, bear down, tune in, and feel my baby make her way closer to meeting me.

As each subsequent contraction passed, I would slow my breath and try to listen to Brian's encouraging words: "good; slow, deep breaths, send some air to our baby; good."

Each time I slowed my breathing, though, I could feel her slip back a little. It was difficult to feel that loss of ground, but also motivating to get some of it back with each contraction that followed. We proceeded like this for what felt like the longest time. At some point, our second midwife arrived. She started listening to baby's heart tones every so often between and sometimes during pushing. Someone kept a cold washcloth on my neck and a straw with coconut water at my mouth. As pushing progressed, our midwife asked if I could change positions a few times. Reluctantly, I did and each time it felt awful and then suddenly I was relieved to be using my leg muscles in a different way. Finally, I could no longer feel her head slipping back when contractions ended, and I was soon instructed to sit back. Two or three strong pushes later, sweet relief washed over me as her head was born, followed shortly by her shoulders and body. Brian played the role of assistant baby catcher and placed our beautiful little girl, Lucia, on my chest at 9:06 p.m.

I feel so incredibly grateful to have had the birth experience I had. It was the single greatest, most magical thing I've ever done. I feel like a different person in many ways, not only because this experience is what made me a mother, but also because it changed the fundamental way I think about myself. I am a warrior; strong and confident and capable of so much more than I ever thought possible! And I'm blessed to have been surrounded and held in the loving arms of my fabulous birth team: my husband who was the guiding voice and strength I needed through the entire process; my doula who held my space, anticipated my silent needs, and kept Brian comfortable; and my midwives who made me feel safe, prepared, capable, and empowered. I cannot thank them all enough!

June Holiday

○ ○ ○ ○ ○ ○ ○ ○ ○ ○ ○ ○ ○ ○ ○ ○ ○ ○

"Based on our decision to birth at home, some people actually assume we don't believe in our kids wearing glasses, going to the dentist, or donning underwear."

—Natalie, stay-at-home mama
San Jose, California

It was March 23rd, and I had just relaxed into bed, feeling myself drift off, when I thought I felt my water break. I reached down between my legs to cup it before I wet the bed—it didn't help much. Like a monkey, I brought my hand to my nose to test the odor and could almost smell my baby's sweet head. The predicted due date was the 25th. I smiled drowsily and staggered blindly toward the bathroom while calling to Justin, who was sound asleep.

I told him, "We're gonna have this baby soon. Like, probably a day early."

Oh, how naive I was.

He didn't quite understand, and kept mumbling from his sleepy state, "Wah? Wah happen?"

I repeated myself several times before it really sunk in (or until he really woke up). By the time, I dried myself and returned to the bedroom, he was sitting straight up in bed, animatedly grinning from ear to ear. I warned him we had to get our butts back to bed; that we would need all the energy we could get. We were in for the long haul now. Like, eighteen plus years, probably. I slept like a log on a pile of towels and dreamed of the ocean and large whales.

The following morning, contractions were a breeze. I was excited and truly looking forward to active labor. (Oooh, how naive.) We went about our day and knocked out the "early labor activity list" we created in Birthing from Within (our favorite home birth childbearing class for first timers). We went grocery shopping and took a long walk. I knitted, I baked a birthday cake, I lounged naked in my backyard. No progress. I journaled, I meditated, I listened to soft rock. No progress. I bounced, I shook, I shouted, I marched up and down the stairs, I listened to hard rock. No progress! The baby did not come on the 24th. The baby did not come on the 25th. Our birth team had come and gone, but the baby had not. I felt like I was being punished for not finishing the nursery in time. The walls were painted, but there wasn't a single piece of furniture in it (still co-sleeping, one year strong). When our midwife had finally checked me the morning of the 25th, we had determined that my water was, in fact, intact. It had probably sprung a leak and resealed. I was only two centimeters dilated. We felt discouraged and very tired. Little did we know that my contractions were steadily gaining force, and our child was entirely prepared to blow this joint.

By that evening, I was in full, active labor. Justin massaged my back, swayed with me in bed, and hummed through each surge. He showered me with kisses and kept my hair out of my face. He said very little, but was my rock all along. We were working together as a team. I fell deeper in love with my husband in the throes of labor than ever before: more than our six-year courtship, more than our one year of marriage. He helped me feel confident. Never once did he doubt my capacity to give birth to our baby at home.

Just moments after midnight on the 26th, I was mentally preparing myself for a hospital transfer. I was beyond exhausted. Contractions were close, and I was falling asleep in between them while sitting on the toilet, buck naked. I remember vividly rocking with Justin on the lip of our tub, waiting for it to fill, and nodding off into him. He wrapped his arms around me to keep me from slamming into the tile. Every break my body allowed me, I felt the grasp of sleep tightening around my looped-out brain. When I finally got in the water, there was so much relief. I would doze here and there in the soothing bath, waking up only to moan through another contraction. Around 3:00 a.m., I was wigging out. There was no more relief. I couldn't find a comfortable position. There was no more escaping this battle. The tug-o-war marathon began. Any thoughts of a hospital transfer vacated my mind, and all I could do was bear witness to the process. I surrendered to my body and to my baby.

To my husband, surrendering sounded a lot like a siren going off in our small master bathroom. I howled like I was possessed. I made noises I didn't know I could make. I scared the shit out of Justin, and probably the neighbors, too. I even scared myself. I started feeling like a huge, violently shaking cave, with wind screaming through its chambers. I was rolling my hips in the water and holding my vagina, making huge swells of water on either side of the tub. Then I felt my water break. It was no leak this time. It burst through my fingers and surged into the tub like the mouth of a great river. I shouted to Justin in both excitement and fear, and he burst through the bathroom door to agree that it had indeed broken. The tub had turned a pale yellow and was a bloody show. Swirling freely in the water were hundreds of tiny white clusters that looked like butter. I picked one up and squished it between my fingers. It was vernix, and I knew things just got real.

Sure enough, as soon as the waters broke, my body took over completely. I felt great, powerful, thrust-like sensations running down my spine, pushing and molding baby down my canal; I couldn't stop it if I tried. My lower body lifted out of the tub, and I knew this child was ready to meet us. In an instant, Justin was on the phone with our midwife, and, much to our relief, she was on her way. However, our midwife misheard Justin's name and rushed over to Rustin's house, whose wife was due the same day as us, and who had also amazingly gone into labor that day; we both delivered our little ones just hours apart. When things got sorted out, and the midwives started arriving, we were almost plus-one. I could feel the baby's head in my vagina; my body was well on its way to shimmying this kid out.

I noticed the sky outside my bathroom window had begun to lighten. I pushed with all my might, wanting so badly to meet my little morning glory. I pushed until my lips turned purple. With every push, the baby's head would emerge and then retreat again. That was the hardest part. I felt myself widening until I didn't think I could anymore.

I kept saying "No more, no more!"

My midwife lovingly responded, "Well, you want to hold your baby, don't you?"

That was all I needed. *Of course, I did!* Yes, more, yes, more! I felt the head emerge and I remember caressing the curly thick locks of my nearly born baby's sweet hair. The hair was just like I imagined it would be. I had been dreaming about it for so long.

My little one torpedoed through the water like a baby whale. Our midwife caught our little water creature and laid our baby on my chest. I cradled the child protectively over my breast, cupping the tiny head in my hand. Everything around me became a blur as my new life's focus lay heaving with me in my tub.

"Oh, my baby, oh, my baby," I kept saying as the child made soft newborn grunts and mews. "I know, baby. That was so hard. But you did such a good job."

I'm not sure if I was talking to myself or my baby. Maybe both of us. Justin kissed us both and I could see the proud gleam of a new daddy in his eyes. He'd been waiting for this moment since he was a child. We basked in these glorious feelings for a good six or seven minutes before we realized we didn't know our child's gender! We counted fingers and toes long before we even remembered to see who we were holding.

I lifted the baby from my chest and announced so very proudly, "It's a girl!"

I think I knew that all along. We named her June Holiday, the Roman protector of women. One day she's going to birth her own as powerfully and as confidently as I did her, and I'll forever recount the day of her birth as an honest-to-goodness holiday. The day we became a family.

Chapter 2

There Has to Be a Better Way: Home Birth after Hospital Birth

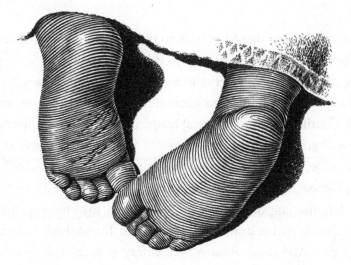

A Rockstar Birth

○ ○ ○ ○ ○ ○ ○ ○ ○ ○ ○ ○ ○ ○ ○ ○ ○

"I did it! I did it at home! I did it on my terms! And I rocked it!
—Shalome, founder of *Rockstar Birth* magazine
Melbourne, Australia

These are the feelings that filter back to me when I think about the home birth of our son, Charlie Reuben. This is his birth journey.

After an unexpectedly intervention-heavy first birth, I knew I wanted a different experience when I next became pregnant. At twenty-weeks pregnant with Charlie, I went to the local hospital, and during the appointment with the midwife-on-duty, I said to her, "I would like to come in here as late as possible, have my baby, and go home as soon as possible." In that moment, I knew this home birthing gig was for me.

As I left that appointment, I quickly called my chiropractor (who's partner recently had a home birth), grabbed his midwife's details, and made the call. And these amazing midwifery women were goddesses in female form. I immediately felt at ease and knew that I wanted to birth at home with them. Forging a relationship with my midwives was one of the highlights of my birth journey. I looked forward to those appointments with glee, not just because we would check the baby's heartbeat or do the fundal height, but because I felt so connected with them. They created a circle where I felt safe and trusted in my ability to birth. We talked about anything and everything, and in doing so, all of my fears about birth were faced and embraced. They truly made my home birth experience something special.

My midwife team also made my family feel ready for birth. They met with my man, our daughter, and my sister (who would be there for our daughter) and made sure that their questions were answered and that they felt comfortable and connected to the experience.

When I told my man that I wanted to birth at home, he said, "oookay." He was very supportive of wherever I wanted to birth (but later confided that he had wondered if he would have to paint the walls and change the carpets afterward).

I immersed myself in positive birth stories and educated myself about the process of labor; I wanted to know every detail. In choosing to birth at home, I was taking responsibility for my own birth, and I wanted to be educated and informed. My man and I undertook a Calm Birth preparation class, which was gold. Not only did it reaffirm the beauty of birth, the class provided me with several tools to birth my baby: breathing techniques, affirmations, visualizations, and meditations. The class also gave my man an incredible insight into what he could do to support me. Suddenly he had a clear role, and he understood how the birth would likely unfold, and which tools he could bring to the table. He was no longer scared of home birth.

As I moved past my "guess date," I started doing some labor acupuncture to encourage our babe to join us. During my second appointment at 41+1, I asked my traditional Chinese medicine (TCM) practitioner to crank it up a bit. I was beyond ready. I was pumped, and I wanted to meet our baby! When I went to bed that evening, there were no serious signs of impending labor, yet I woke bolt upright with a strong contraction at midnight. I tried to lie back down and see if I could fall asleep and another came like a train. No sleeping for me!

I went out to the couch to see if there was some rhythm and regularity to my surges. I didn't want to call my midwives in case it wasn't the real deal, so I spent two hours timing contractions, listening to my meditation music, and getting into my groove. Around 2:00 a.m., my man came out and I asked him to start timing the contractions. In handing that over and no longer having to think anymore, I immediately dropped deep into labor land. I was able to let go; to release and surrender.

I heard my man call the midwives about twenty minutes later.

He whispered, "Her surges are three minutes apart and last for one minute."

I remember thinking *really? Fantastic! That means we're on!* In that moment, I had no concept of time and space; it was so affirming to know that we were progressing beautifully.

About thirty minutes later, my midwives gently bustled in and touched me on the arm. I had experienced some bleeding with my surges, so my midwife asked if it would be okay for her to do an internal exam, and I immediately consented. Lying down on my back wasn't comfortable, but I trusted my midwife. I trusted everything she did and said. I felt so respected and loved as I laid on that bed.

After checking my cervix, she said, "Everything is great. You are great. Your baby is great, and you're seven centimeters."

I was ecstatic! Her positive language and demeanor helped me stay in my birthing zone. My midwives encouraged me to get upright and use gravity to help my baby descend. For the next couple of hours, I labored with my man over the kitchen table while the midwives waited in the next room, gifting us space to birth together. I was craving heat on my lower back, so he passed me heat packs from the microwave while keeping me hydrated with water. It was starting to get intense, and I was starting to get really vocal with long, slow, deep moans (like a cow).

After one particularly long surge, I recall hearing my midwife from the doorway saying, "Ooh, just listen to that. That is the sound of a woman bringing her baby down beautifully."

I thought, *f*ck yeah, I really am!*

Her words gave me that surge of womb power to keep going.

While timing my contractions before the midwives arrived, my man had filled up a massive pool in the lounge room. I was getting my hippy chick on and totally thought that I would want to birth in the water. As my labor was progressing, I was looking for different positions to bring relief. My midwives asked if I wanted to get in the big, deep pool. Ah, no. Sorry, Lover, but I had changed my mind. I wanted heat on my lower back. Lots of heat, and the pool just wasn't going to cut it. Instead, I headed into the shower (where I had spent immense amounts of my time meditating on my birth during pregnancy) and spent the next forty-five minutes roaring through my surges with the shower water drumming on my lower back.

It was about 5:30 a.m. now, and as birth was getting closer, our six-year-old daughter, Scarlett, woke up. I remember seeing her face pushed up against the shower glass, as questions came pouring out of her sleeping head: "What are you doing, mummy? Can I get in with you? Why are you moaning like that? Will the baby slip down the plug hole? Can I have some toast?" I was laughing between contractions and chatting to her as much as possible. My sister woke up, too, and spent time preparing Scarlett for the birth by rereading her favorite birth books, reminding her of the noises and sights that would likely come soon, and making cups of tea for the midwives.

Then my darling midwife asked, "Do you want to have your baby in the shower?"

I was so vague and smiley that I replied, "I don't know, do I? Where else could I go?"

She said, "Why don't you come out on the couch?"

Again, without question, I went to the lounge room where my team had made a beautiful nest of blankets for me. On all fours, I crawled onto the nest, and breathed our baby down. With my man by my head, and my daughter and sister watching the baby, I used all of my incredible womb energy, all of the positive and empowering stories I had read, all of the energy of the women who had birthed before me, the strength and love via my man's hands, and I breathed that baby out.

Our baby was passed through my legs, up onto my chest, and I was helped onto my back.

I snuggled down with him, and I gazed at my man (who was crying), and said, "Oh, wow, it's a baby! How amazing! Look at that."

In my moment of awe, I hadn't yet thought to check the gender. We have three daughters between us, so when Scarlett leaned over and announced that we had a boy, I was so freaking ecstatic.

Charlie Reuben had joined our family.

This birth made me so high. It was the most spectacular moment of my life. And I don't mean just because I was now holding our baby; new babies are so cool, but I mean the actual birth. I felt so incredibly fulfilled about how I had done it, about who I had done it with. I felt like I had worked on a nine-month project, not just nourishing our baby in my womb, but preparing myself for this birthing moment. I had done it! I had called in the team, my man and I made sure we felt ready, we had my sister and daughter there—it was lush! I have never felt more feminine, more powerful, more voluptuous, more sensual. When I breathed that baby down, I felt like a warrior—like a Rockstar. Every woman deserves to feel like that in birth, no matter how or where her journey unfolds. We all deserve to know that birth can be so incredibly positive, powerful, and transformative.

It's official. I am addicted to home birth. And if I can do it, so can you. You've got this, mama. Everything you need is already inside you.

Rekita in Georgia

○ ○ ○ ○ ○ ○ ○ ○ ○ ○ ○ ○ ○ ○ ○ ○ (○

"I was able to have my family and my kids around without having to accommodate others. I was comfortable. I labored my way, without judgment for being nude or too loud."

—Rekita, homemaker and childcare provider
Atlanta, Georgia

After six births, I was finally going to try home birth with my seventh babe. I always wanted to have a home birth and water birth, but I was a little scared. When Angelina, my midwife, said that she would be taking on home births, I got excited.

When I went into her office and the staff asked, "Rekita, are you going to do a home birth," I didn't know how to answer.

So, I ran the idea by my husband, and he was down for it. Once I knew my husband was supportive of us having a home birth, it was an easy answer: *yes!*

My mom was skeptical about the whole home birth idea and started asking all the usual questions: "what if this?" and "what if that?" I just think she wanted to make sure we would be okay. My home birth would be a first for my midwife, Angelina, and, of course, a first for me, too. However, my hospital experiences with my first six labors were not great, and I was sure I didn't want to go through another hospital birth. While birthing my sixth child, my labor stopped and had to be started again. While waiting, a doctor on staff told my midwife at the time that she could go home, and that she would deliver my son via Cesarean. From that point on, I said I would not go back to that hospital. I also knew how I wanted to labor. During labor, I get very hot. Hospitals frown on walking around nude, but at home I could do just that and be comfortable. I wanted to be able to walk to the park by my house and dance freely without being hooked up to noisy monitors. Like I said, choosing home birth with Angelina was an easy choice.

I went into labor with our home birth babe during my maternity photo shoot, and Angelina was already there.

Angelina jokingly asked, "Rekita, am I going to have to set up the pool today?"

Sure enough, the first stages of labor had begun, and I was three centimeters dilated. Once my contractions started, we started getting everything set up for the birth. Suddenly, my labor stopped.

Not being upset or disappointed, Angelina said, "I will see you next time."

A couple of days later, the contractions started back up again. Angelina and I walked, laughed, and talked about how next time we should go to the beach for me to deliver. Angelina even went to the store while my hubby and I tried some natural ways to increase my contractions, but they stopped again.

Third time was a charm! On May 10th, Angelina had come over to check on me after I lost my mucus plug the previous night. She stripped my membranes and my contractions picked up immediately. I started walking and dancing through the contractions. Around 7:00 p.m. Angelina broke my water and my labor continued to progress.

At about 8:55 p.m., my body became very calm and Angelina asked, "Are you ready to get in the water?"

I said, "No."

She asked again, and I decided to try the pool. Angelina told me to use the bathroom first. As I did, I let out a loud groan. Angelina knew it was time to push, and she ushered me into the birthing pool. I got into the birthing pool and experienced one contraction. With the second contraction, I pushed out my daughter, Zephaniah Inara Bradley. It was 9:18 p.m.; we were surrounded by her siblings, my doula, Delandra, Angelina's assistant, and my mom's best friend, Lakeya.

After I got out of the birthing pool, I went to my room, where my four-year-old son cut his sister's umbilical cord. After that, my daughter was weighed and measured. Lakeya gave my daughter her first bath while I rested in bed. Delandra made the call for my placenta to be picked up to be capsuled. Angelina came and checked on me and baby twenty-four hours later. She came back forty-eight hours later and did baby's blood screening and newborn photos. We never had to leave our home . . . or beds!

The birth went so smoothly. I would do it all over again. Angelina waited patiently while my labor progressed; I had no pressure to hurry up. I never felt like I had to rush because someone needed the room. My doula and Angelina's assistant treated me wonderfully. Even though it took three days for me to deliver, it didn't matter. Angelina was there every step of the way: from the beginning with home visits and pregnancy photos to newborn checkups and photos.

I had never felt this great after a delivery. All I wanted after the delivery of my child was to sleep; I was able to have that with home birth. I love the fact that Angelina made me feel special. I wish I'd had all my babies at home. There is nothing like waking up with your baby and being comfortable without your sleep being interrupted. With having a home birth, I could birth wherever I wanted: the living room, bedroom, bathroom, my back porch under the stars, anywhere.

Birthing at home meant I could do the things I wanted and needed to do while in labor. I was able to interact with my kids, FaceTime my other midwife, and, most importantly, laugh and have fun with my friends. My midwife, Angelina, was the best. She kept me laughing through the pain. She let my body do what it was supposed to do to bring my daughter into this world. I was able to be open, be loud, and stay calm. I was able to have my family and my kids around without having to accommodate others. I was comfortable. I labored *my* way, without judgment for being nude or too loud. I was able to eat a home-cooked meal. I was able to sleep in my own bed and my baby in hers. It was the birth I had wanted. I enjoyed having a home birth so much that we are currently working on having another home birth soon!

Fear and Triumph

○ ○ ○ ○ ○ ○ ○ ○ ○ ○ ○ ○ ○ ○ ○ ○ ○ ○

"Fear. This is how I approached every other labor up until now. It's been a few days since my daughter was born, and I can't believe I'm standing in the same shower I labored in. As the hot water washes away the past few days, I reflect on how every room in our home will always hold some amazing aura from the day my baby was born."

—Diane, author and illustrator

Taylor, Michigan

I can't pinpoint when labor started, but it felt like I was in labor for days. I was due on Friday, April 22nd, and by that night I was feeling overwhelmingly discouraged. Since the last pregnancy had ended in a miscarriage, I feared that anything could go wrong, to the point that I had trouble bonding with my unborn baby until the sixth or seventh month of pregnancy. That Friday, I confided in my husband about my deep fear of no baby. My husband reacted, "Don't even say that!" I felt that his words meant I could jinx our baby, and I began to cry for hours. I achingly wanted this baby, and I didn't trust it would come to fruition. The next day, Saturday, I met with my midwife; it was such a good visit. She happened to be by herself, and she calmed all my fears. She reassured me that my feelings were normal and okay. She recommended an outing and some fun with the family. When she left, I felt much better and we ventured out to Elizabeth Park for a walk.

I had mild and irregular contractions that Saturday night. I called my midwife, hoping this was the real thing, but they were far from lasting a minute and were not yet five minutes apart, so I was told to call back when they were. I fell asleep shortly after and awoke in the morning feeling great.

At this point, I was overdue by two days and afraid I would never actually go into labor, much less deliver a live baby.

On Sunday afternoon, I decided we should go bowling to induce labor. The midwife did say to get active, and throwing heavy balls at pins seemed like a good way to jumpstart labor! It seemed to work, as contractions started up and lasted throughout dinner and into the evening. I went to bed with the contractions continuing, waking me up almost every hour. The contractions were intense, yet bearable. The next morning, the contractions seemed to come and go. I called my good friend, Rachael, to compare notes, as she had delivered three babies since I delivered my last one. After talking to Rachael, who had been two weeks overdue with her last baby, I was convinced that this was going to be two weeks of prodromal labor for me, too. My contractions would come every ten minutes or so, and then they would be farther apart and weaker. Then, nothing at all. My mom hung out and watched TV with me that Monday. At around noon, I decided to straighten up the boys' room. I had been sitting on the floor, organizing clothes for a while, when I tried to stand up, resulting in the most painful contraction yet. I breathed through it and decided that my mom and I should go for a walk.

The contractions got extremely painful when I was on my feet, but I was determined to get up and move. We made it out of the house, but I barely made it to the end of the street before I suggested we walk home; the contractions were just too painful standing up. After we walked home, it was lunchtime, so my mom took me to Taco Bell. I mean, you've gotta eat and keep up your energy! My mom drove, as I couldn't drive safely through a contraction, should one come. As we were waiting to pay in the drive thru, I sat in the passenger seat breathing through a contraction. My contractions were regularly irregular, so I had hope.

Once we got home and ate, I sat on my birthing ball, all the while using an app on my phone to keep track of the contractions. My mom kept urging me to contact the midwife, but my contractions weren't lasting a minute at five minutes apart, and it seemed like I'd be jumping the gun. By 3:30 p.m., I figured I'd call Rob home from work. (I'd told him to go because earlier in the morning I was convinced I'd be pregnant for another two weeks.) The contractions were now lasting anywhere from thirty to fifty seconds and increasing in intensity. Soon the contractions were strong and coming every three minutes. Much to my mom's relief, we promptly called the midwife, too. Rob was home by 4:00 p.m., and it was evident that this was *it*; I was in labor. As soon as Rob arrived, he got busy filling the birth pool.

The next three hours were a whirlwind. I suddenly started worrying that the midwives wouldn't come soon enough. They arrived at 5:30 p.m., and I breathed a sigh of relief; their advice was like gold, and I did whatever they suggested.

The first time I got out of the tub was to pee. They never rushed me, and let me go at my own pace. I vividly remember their tender care as they helped take off my purple dress, and dry me, as well. It was like the movies I had seen where all the matriarchs come together to care for the new mom. It was lovely in all its intensity. I moved at a snail's pace between contractions, thriving in the relaxing atmosphere of my home. Linda, the head midwife, asked to check me.

I replied, "Sure, I just swear I better be more than two centimeters."

She laughed, hoping the results wouldn't deter me. I laid on the couch in the living room.

"You are four centimeters," she said, "and your bag of waters is bulging."

She barely finished her statement before my water broke. There was a break in the contractions for a few minutes, and it was sweet relief. I knew that things were progressing in a timely fashion. I made my way back to the tub, and the contractions intensified. My best friend-turned-doula became such a help at this stage, talking me through my contractions with her ten-month-old strapped to her back and my husband putting pressure on my back. They were the dream team I didn't know I would need or so heavily rely on.

My contractions were getting stronger and closer together. One of the midwives suggested that since I liked the birthing tub, I should try a different position in the shower to help with the pain I was feeling. As I moved to the shower, I felt this tension between my body and the birthing process. I tried to relax my body to make each contraction count, but a part of me was afraid I would rip open. Letting myself squat seemed impossible. I made it to the toilet after 20 minutes in the shower, as the midwives suggested. I labored through a few contractions on the toilet and then made my way downstairs where the birthing stool was set up in the living room. The midwives were eating and they laughed because they had gone into the living room to avoid bothering me with their food. I didn't care. Suddenly I was sitting comfortably, as comfortable as one could be that far along in labor, on this amazing birthing stool. The pillows were stacked up in front of me as I faced the couch, and my body relaxed into the cushions as I tried to succumb to the contractions. I kept telling myself, *I'm not gonna die, I can do this.*

Everyone kept telling me how great I was doing, but I felt the full wrath of my body being slowly pulled open from the inside, like arms and legs being pulled apart in a medieval torture device. I clung to their words, not fully believing them, knowing the only way out of the pain was through it. What looked like peaceful moaning in labor felt like chaos from the inside.

In the moments when I was in second stage labor, the pain was unbearable. In all my agony and concentration, I would have done anything that was asked of me. I could not have advocated for myself effectively. How easy it would have been in a hospital for the wrong nurse to convince me into unnecessary medication or intervention. At the peak of my surges I lamented my home birth choice, but the regret was fleeting with every moment. I knew I was in good hands and that I was capable of birthing my baby.

With every surge, I chanted "Just one at a time, just one at a time."

I clung to the words my doula whispered in my ear as my husband pressed firmly on my back: "It's going to reach a peak, and then it's going to start fading away."

I clung to her words even when the surges piggybacked and the pain barely waned.

I heard Rachael's voice again, "Every surge brings you closer to your baby."

All I could think was that there could be a hundred contractions left or a thousand; was I a mile or just a millimeter closer? I clung to her words in the unknown. The only fear here was the fear of time passing. How much longer? I clung to the side of the birthing pool, trying to release every muscle in my body.

I began to feel nauseous, and I threw up. The head midwife was in the background telling me it's a good sign, that the baby would be born soon.

I thought to myself, *does that mean any minute, soon? Or in like, ten minutes, soon? How soon is soon?*

Heather, one of the midwives, was on my right, and Rachael was on my left. Rob was a presence that worked by my side, yet in the background. I imagine Linda, the head midwife, as the godfather—nay, godmother—of the goings on in the room: sitting in the black armchair, overseeing it all with her notebook. I was told to push whenever I felt like it, so I rode each wave praying for that urge to push; to birth my baby. Suddenly, I felt a creeping pressure, but it was not the pressure I was expecting.

"I think I have to push," I said. "Tell my mom and Bobbie (Rob's mom) they can come up!"

With the next contraction, I began to push. The ring of fire was not the burn I was expecting, though I felt I might split open at any moment.

Vaguely remembering the doctor's assistance in every previous birth, I asked, "Can't you pull her out?"

Linda replied in a matter-of-fact tone, "No, hun, you're gonna have to push her out."

Push her out I did, and she plopped on the floor through the birthing stool. Sweet relief! In hindsight, it seemed very hazy in a surreal sort of way. Heather was calling my name to take my baby from beneath the birthing stool, but I felt like I couldn't move. I did grab my baby from below, her umbilical cord attached to the placenta still inside me.

What do I do? I wondered.

I could feel everything and I couldn't comprehend the feeling of the umbilical cord hanging out from within, still attached to the little person in my arms that I never thought would come. I remember most vividly, the swirl of blond on the crown of her head, and reveling in the relief. The full capacity of my daughter's birth didn't really sink in until the next day.

Sitting here staring at my baby girl, I am so happy I had my baby at home. I knew what was best before I was in distress, and I could never have fought the system at the hospital. When I was in labor, I remember taking every suggestion from the midwives because I figured they knew more than I did and I would have done anything to relieve the pain of each surge. The relieving pressure of my husband's hands on my lower back made the pain easier to bare. No matter where he went, when a contraction came, he was right there as soon as I called. I could hear his hip-hopping steps coming to my rescue. Knowing he was there was beyond comforting. It was the constant reminder that I wasn't going through this alone. When Rachael, my best friend and doula, talked me through each contraction, telling me that it would peak and wane, I clung to that reaffirmation. Though I knew her words to be true, I had to hear them over and over again.

While on that birthing stool I remember telling myself, *you are not gonna die, this isn't going to kill you.*

I was trying to calm my fear of the pain, because it felt like death was the only option, when in fact, life, the birth of a new baby, was the only option to relieve the pain.

My first shower after having the baby, I stared at the walls inside the bath tub, remembering the time I spent leaning against the tiles, breathing through each contraction. My home holds the memories of the most peaceful birth I've ever experienced. Yvette Arya Christine Grove is my fourth baby. She is a blessed rainbow baby and miracle after the loss of our Hannah during our last pregnancy.

My mother-in-law has been a nurse for many years. After witnessing this beautiful event, she is a convert to the home birth way of life. She witnessed Yvette born into such peace and love that she says she could never see it done any other way. Our home is truly blessed!

Samyra

○ ○ ○ ○ ○ ○ ○ ○ ○ ○ ○ ○ ○ ○ ○ ○ ○ ○

"The most important aspect of my home birth was that I was able to experience my birth, my way. There was no one there saying, 'you cannot.' My birth team only said, 'you can.' As simple as it seems, that in itself was an honor!"

—Samyra, licensed massage therapist
Georgia

After two prior "tryouts" for labor, I decided to get walking in an effort to get labor started for real! I walked many times around the playground, up a high flight of steps, around our local mall, and on a three-mile trail that ended with me picking up the pace around the perimeter of the park; I was determined. Finally, my body decided it was time for "the real thing!" Contractions were about three minutes apart, and I was sweating more from all the walking than from the contractions!

We headed back home where I planned to sew clothes for the little one, as, quite frankly, I wasn't convinced I was in labor. I suppose I was in denial, but I didn't want to call the midwife until I was one hundred percent sure that the contraction wouldn't fizzle out; it didn't take long!

Within thirty minutes of being home from our three-mile walk, the first smack of reality came. I quickly took a deep breath and mentally said, "you got this." Soon after, I got onto all fours and held onto the exercise ball through each breath. At this point I knew these were good contractions, but breathing on all fours soon stopped being cute or masking the discomfort.

I told my husband I needed to get in the shower. Now, I'm not sure what happened, but when I got into the bedroom, it got real. I immediately undressed. The contractions were getting a little more than intense, but they were not overwhelming. My husband tells this part of the story a bit differently than I do. As a matter of fact, he asked how I was going from making faces of pain right back to the conversation we were having!

My husband asked if I wanted to call our midwife, and I remember barely getting out "not yet." He asked if I was sure before stepping out. Little did I know, he and my mother decided to call the midwife anyway. I got out of the shower and he talked me through the following contractions that were pretty official. He told me they called our midwife, but he was going to call her again because now the contractions were around 90 seconds apart.

It was nutz! Yes, nutz with a z.

My husband was telling me, "Aight Babe, you have about fifteen seconds. Aight Babe, we have ten seconds before another hits. Let's get this on you."

Upon reflection, I was so appreciative because he let me grab his chest, arms, and hands when I felt I couldn't stand. He took the time to tend to me while my body was preparing for baby. Okay, enough sappy stuff.

I never got dressed; there was no point! The contractions needed all of our attention. We had clothes picked out that we wanted to labor in, but all of that went out the window when our midwives arrived.

I remember our midwife, Angelina, saying something like, "Oh yea, we have a baby on the way."

I was mid-contraction and making a "Flavor Flav face" as my husband so hilariously describes it. Angelina came in to check my cervix per request. I was curious. I was six centimeters, but I would have guessed eight! Nonetheless, everything moved rapidly from there. I immediately got into the pool and enjoyed its warmth. Then, a contraction! I remember trying to get my entire belly into the water, and once the contraction was done, I leaned over the side of the birth pool. In all honesty, I was tired. I remember saying that I wanted to nap. It went that way with my husband applying ice and everyone watching . . . waiting. This process went on for about forty minutes, but it seemed like mere moments.

I recall my husband and I being face to face on the side of the pool. In each other's space, quietly present, and still. The water masked the intensity

I felt, and then I began to feel nauseous. I verbalized that and they helped me out of the water.

Once in the bathroom, my body did the rest of its cleansing and I got to experience my water breaking for the first time. It was quite a surprise! I wanted my water to break, but I wasn't expecting it in that moment of being sick to my stomach (which was another first). That was a surprise I didn't expect, since I hadn't even experienced one day of morning sickness. Immediately, Angelina said I needed to get back in the water.

My husband joined me in the water and the soon-to-be big sisters held my hands. Right at that moment, it seemed like it was time to push. I remember Angelina saying, "Listen to your body." I remember listening to Jah Cure playing, and it seemed as if he was speaking directly to me. "You're strong enough . . . to reach your destination . . . nothing . . . nothing is impossible." At that moment, I began to push. Angelina told me to stop for a moment. And then she gave me the okay to finish delivering our little one.

To describe the birth of our daughter two months later seems surreal. To put your mind to something and to accomplish it is to "reach your destination." When my husband passed our newly born daughter to me, I was in complete awe. I don't know what else to say besides it was a captivating moment. In the moments where I was pushing, it felt like an out-of-body experience, yet I was very present; like a lucid dream. This birth we so desired had manifested in the most beautiful way, bringing an experience of harmony and joy.

Chapter 3

Just Another Version of Normal

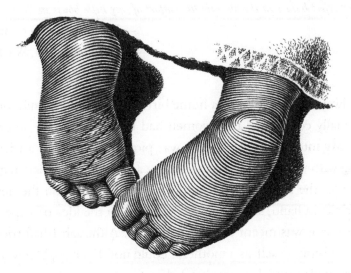

Twins!

o o o o o o o o o o o o o o o o o o

"I had done it! I had labored through the pain of a separated rib and had birthed two completely perfect babies in the warmly lit comfort of my little house in the country."
—Erica, shipping coordinator
Woodland, Washington

I didn't always know I wanted a home birth. It might sound silly, but I had never actually considered that women had babies anywhere other than a hospital. My interest in home birth was piqued in 2009, by a friend who was living with us and studying to become a midwife. Over late night conversations in the kitchen and Saturday afternoon chats on the deck with boozy drinks in hand, she slowly woke me up to the idea of experiencing birth the way it was meant to be experienced. Although I had tried many times to envision myself as a mother, I could not. Even so, I knew it would happen someday, and I knew that I desperately wanted to have a home birth when that day came.

The stories my friend would share, and the home birth narratives I poured over by Ina May Gaskin* spoke of a physical and spiritual transformation, a reaching of the end of one's self and abilities, a surrendering to a deep, primitive power that goes beyond knowledge and desire, the role as a woman to participate with the divine to bring forth life. These stories spoke of womanhood, of partnership, of spirituality, of magic. And I wanted to experience that.

---

*Ina May Gaskin is a highly respected and trusted midwife, author, educator, and founder of the Farm Midwifery Center in Summertown, Tennessee. The Farm was founded in 1971 and has seen the births of nearly 3,000 babies.

In July of 2014, my husband and I had a talk that went something like, "Well, it's now or never!" And we decided to start our family. When my husband was sixteen, he was paralyzed in a car accident and became a C6/C7 quadriplegic. Because of this, our only option for conception was through in vitro fertilization. We began the long and grueling process in August 2014, and I became pregnant with twins on December 7th. After having confirmed that both embryos were thriving, I excitedly called the midwife that I had chosen for my home birth months before I became pregnant. My husband and I met with her when I was nine weeks along, and there was an instant connection. She was so comforting and encouraging and seemed thrilled to have the opportunity to work with us and deliver the babies. She drew my blood and sent me on my way. About a week later, she called to tell me that my blood panel looked great, but that she was unable to be my midwife. She had discussed the birth with her team and they did not feel like it would be wise to take me on as a patient. They felt uncomfortable attending a twin birth because it was too high risk. I was shocked. Maybe I should have anticipated this, but I suppose that's not the way my mind is wired. I figured birthing two babies wasn't any different than birthing one; it was just another variation of normal. But I quickly figured out that it isn't viewed that way in the hospital medical model or in the majority of midwifery communities.

After being turned down by our first midwife, I spent the next four weeks searching for a way to get the birth I wanted. I talked to countless midwives on the phone who all told me the same thing: it's just too risky. I even called The Farm Midwifery Center (a home birth–centered community in Tennessee where you can live in a cabin and birth your babies next to a warm fire or a babbling brook or wherever you please).

They told me, "No, sorry, we don't do twins for first-time mothers. Your pelvis has not been tried and proven true."

Feeling totally discouraged, I scheduled my first prenatal appointment with a doctor at the hospital.

Not being a big fan of conventional medicine, I had just bounced around between a number of different naturopaths over the years, so I did not have a primary care physician or obstetrician (OB). A midwifery clinic in the area recommended a doctor who had proven to be less intervening than most regarding multiples. I was scared to death going into that appointment. Through all the research I'd done over the last four weeks, I'd come to realize that if I thought having a single baby in the hospital had the potential for too much intervention, it was much worse with multiples. I also realized that in all the stories I had read about home birth, I'd never come across a story about twins.

At my first prenatal appointment, the nurse practitioner had me on my back with my legs apart, performing a PAP before I even knew what was happening. In the back of my mind, I thought, *wait, isn't this one of the things I'm supposed to* not *be letting them do?* She then began quizzing me on which vaccines I was current on and which ones I planned to get while pregnant. I told her I had to think about it. On the drive home, I pictured a long and difficult path ahead of me, with the end result being quite different than what I had always dreamed of. I felt stuck. I felt controlled. I felt confused about why I couldn't have the birth I wanted. My deepest desire was to do what was best for my babies, but everyone was making me feel like the thing I thought was best was actually the worst.

Two weeks later I received a letter in the mail from the hospital stating that I had tested positive for Group B strep. I wasn't sure what that meant so I started doing some research. During the next twenty weeks of research and reflection, I began to put together what this birth might look like. They were going to want to induce at thirty-eight weeks. If I refused induction, I would be required to come in for non-stress tests twice a week for the remaining two weeks. If I actually made it to forty weeks, then I would need to be induced immediately. I would need IV antibiotics during labor and continuous fetal monitoring. I would not be able to get in the water, and I would not be able to move around at all since I would be hooked up to so many things. I could labor in a delivery room, but I would be required to transition to the operating room and deliver on the operating table. I could refuse an epidural, but it was highly likely that the anesthesiologist would want to insert the catheter into my spine anyway, just in case a C-section needed to happen. I was told that the babies could very likely need to go immediately to the NICU. Forget about delayed cord-clamping. As I drew near the thirty-six-week mark, the birth began to weigh heavily on my heart. I started to become quite distressed. And then three things happened that changed the course of everything.

A friend contacted me on Facebook and told me that a friend of hers had just had twins at home. She gave me the names of the midwives that had delivered her babies. Two days later, a different friend told me about these same midwives and encouraged me to call them. A few days after that, I went to my parents' house to soak my aching body in their six-foot bathtub, and my mom left me a newspaper article about home birth to read. I decided to take action. I climbed out of the tub and called the midwife, Mary. I said, "Hi, this might sound crazy, but I'm thirty-six weeks pregnant with twins and I really want to switch to a home birth." She assured me it didn't sound crazy and asked me to come in and talk to her, so I made an appointment for the next day. As my husband and I chatted with Mary and her daughter, Pita, in their cozy, wood-paneled office, I began to feel at ease in a way that I hadn't felt throughout my entire pregnancy. We decided to move forward with a home birth. I was ecstatic. I called my doctor and explained that I would be leaving his care to have my babies at home. He was so supportive! I couldn't believe it. He said he had attended many home births, and he thought they were a beautiful thing. He said I was the perfect candidate. He gave me his pager number and told me to page him if he could walk my midwives through anything or if he could pave the way to the hospital in case I needed to be transported. He wished me luck. And just like that, I was free to bring these babies into the world the best way I saw fit.

The next few weeks were exciting. Mary brought the birth tub up to our house. Did I mention we live WAY out in the country? Like, no cell service out there! It was August, so we inflated the tub on our deck and filled it with cold water. I spent many an afternoon lounging in the sun. As my due date approached, I began to wonder what the beginning signs of labor would feel like. I felt like I was going to be pregnant forever. The morning of my due date, I woke up and just knew these babies were not going to come anytime soon. As the days dragged on, I began to dread the sound of my phone buzzing with notifications from concerned friends. It felt like everyone, even friends I had not connected with in years, were worried about me, the babies, and my decision to have a home birth. The questions started pouring in.

"You're *how* far along?"

"At what point will your midwives induce you?"

"At what point will they send you to the hospital if you never go into labor?"

Then there were the silent questions that no one was asking, but everyone was thinking. *Aren't you concerned that your placentas might be breaking down? Aren't you worried about stillbirth?* I had been so sure, so confident that I was making the best decision for the babies, to have them at home, but I, too, started to wonder those same questions. Looking back, those last five or six days leading up to the birth were the most mentally challenging times of the whole experience.

Finally, at forty-one weeks pregnant, I decided to make an acupuncture appointment to see if we could get things moving. The morning after my appointment at 3:00 a.m., I woke up to a gush between my legs. Yes! My water is breaking! I rolled out of bed and waddled to the bathroom. Without turning on the light I sat down on the toilet and wiped. I looked at the toilet paper and it was dark. I flipped the light on and saw bright red blood. I told my husband, and we decided to call Mary.

Mary was not concerned, but told me if it would make me feel better, she could send me to the hospital for an ultrasound in the morning. I thanked Mary, put on a pad, and went back to bed. The next morning, my mom and I went to the hospital, and the ultrasound looked great. Both babies were a nice, healthy size and the placentas looked good—everything was okay. The next day was my dad's birthday, and while my husband was at work, I went shopping with my parents. Nothing happened. Two days later, my husband and I went to my parents' house for lunch, and when we came home, I laid down for a nap. I woke up around 5:00 p.m. to my body telling me labor was near. My mood felt serious. My spirit felt grounded. The babies felt low.

My mom sent me a message asking me to send her a picture of my belly. She'd been taking a picture every time she'd seen me for the last two weeks in case it was the last time she saw me before the babies arrived. She'd forgotten to take one at lunch that afternoon. I stood in front of the full-length mirror in my bedroom and snapped a side shot. I noticed in my reflection that my belly seemed very, very low.

That evening, my husband and I cleaned the house from top to bottom. I scrubbed sinks and toilets, vacuumed floors, and dusted window sills. We ate dinner, played two games of cribbage, and went to bed. At 3:00 a.m., I woke to use the bathroom and noticed a sharp twinge of pain on my left-hand side that felt like a rib had separated. I couldn't take a deep breath without pain. I hoped it was just a temporary muscle twinge and went back to sleep. On Sunday morning, the pain was still there, but a little sharper. With my background in massage therapy, I concluded that the babies had moved down and out of my ribs, leaving behind several overstretched ligaments. It made sense as I had been sleeping on my right side in bed with the weight of my belly pulling on the left intercostal muscles and tendons. As a result, a rib had slipped. I think I was in early labor, but all I could focus on was the pain just below my left shoulder blade.

It's a funny thing, delivering at home, because you don't want to call your support team too early, but you definitely don't want to call too late. My doula, Jennifer, lived about an hour away so I didn't want to waste her time and gas for a false alarm. However, as the day turned into night, I was beginning to have a difficult time with the pain in my left rib. In hindsight, I think I was having contractions, but they were triggering such intense muscle spasms around the separated rib that I couldn't feel a rhythm to the pain. Around 10:30 p.m., I told my husband that I didn't feel like I could get through the pain on my own anymore, and asked him to call Jennifer. She is also a massage therapist, and I hoped that she would be able to alleviate some of the pain.

Jennifer arrived around midnight and massaged my back for two hours while I sat on my exercise ball. Finally, at 2:00 a.m., she encouraged us to go to bed and try to get some sleep. I woke at 4:00 a.m. to intense muscle spasms surrounding the rib. I woke her up and told her I wanted to get into the birth tub, hoping the warm water would help the pain. After fifteen minutes in the tub, I realized it wasn't working, and I got out. The next eight hours are a blur. I believe I was in full labor, but I couldn't tell when a contraction started or finished. All I could feel was the searing pain in that mid-thoracic region. I went from the birth tub to the couch to the bed while Jennifer followed me around, massaging my back and catching my vomit in a metal stockpot. My husband began calling every chiropractor in a fifty-mile radius, but nobody was open on Labor Day. Finally, he called my midwife and explained what was going on. She happened to have the cell phone number for a chiropractor whose office was only twenty minutes from us. My husband called him and he answered; he was shopping at Ikea with his wife. He agreed to meet us at his office at noon.

My husband and I drove the twenty minutes to the chiropractor's office while Jennifer stayed behind and caught up on sleep. Sitting on the adjustment table, he asked me which rib was out. I told him if he lifted up my shirt, he'd be able to tell because the whole area was bright red. He palpated the rib, faced me toward him, wrapped me in a huge bear hug, and at forty-two weeks pregnant with twins and in active labor, he laid me down on my back and jumped on top of me. I let out a yell and just like that, the rib was back in. I sat up and took a deep breath, something I had not been able to do since the day before. The area was still sore, but I could breathe, and I was immensely grateful for that. He instructed me to ice the area ten minutes on, ten minutes off for the next few hours and sent me on my way.

We got home at 1:00 p.m., and I laid in bed icing my rib. At 3:00 p.m. I decided I'd had enough. Although the rib was back in place, the contractions were still triggering intense muscle spasms around the traumatized rib. Even though I could now breath through the pain, I felt like I had reached my limit. I told my husband and doula that I wanted to go to the hospital and I wanted an epidural, but I needed to know if it could be placed high enough to numb my entire thoracic spine. I needed this pain gone like yesterday. Jennifer said she didn't think that would be possible. I felt so discouraged. We had not summoned my midwives yet because they did not want to arrive until I was near transition, but I had no idea how far I'd progressed because I hadn't had my cervix checked. I told Jennifer that if my midwives arrived and I was only dilated to a three, we were going to the hospital for sure.

She said, "What if you're dilated to a six?"

"I don't know," I wailed.

I was at a loss. I was physically spent. My brain felt like mush with the flood of hormones and pain. Jennifer calmly encouraged me to lay back down for thirty more minutes. My husband held a new ice pack on my rib, and Jennifer went into the other room to get some rest.

For the next forty-five minutes I felt, for the first time, my contractions come on as waves, one after the other. I audibly groaned through each one and slept in the short spaces between each contraction. My husband followed suit, matching his voice to mine with each groan. Through each wave, he held the ice to my back. During this time together, he managed to text the midwives, asking them to come over. I remember bearing down through two intense contractions and opening my eyes.

I muttered, "How long have we been doing this?"

From the other room, Jennifer called out, "About forty-five minutes, and these contractions have been about a minute long and ninety seconds apart."

"We need to call Mary," I exclaimed.

My husband replied that Mary was already on her way. Mary and Pita arrived about ten minutes later.

Mary came into the bedroom and asked if I'd like her to check my cervix.

"*Yes!*" I almost shouted.

She felt around and told us there was no cervix. Jennifer let out a cry of delight and I burst into tears. She helped me out of bed, the midwives filled the birth tub (for the hundredth time that day), and thirty minutes later I was easing my body into the warm water. After two hours of pushing, I finally felt the fullness and pressure of a little head between my legs. I felt the gush of my waters breaking as Baby A was crowning. I made the conscious decision to relax and allow myself to open. One more push and Baby A was out. It was, by far, the hardest thing I've ever done in my life. The relief was so great that I sat back and closed my eyes. Pita called to me, "Look at your baby." I looked down and saw a squished little face and remembered that I had no idea if it was a boy or a girl. Pita couldn't pull the baby out of the water far enough because the cord was too short so she instructed me to feel between the legs under the water. I hope I never forget the feeling of those little balls in my hands!

"It's a boy" I called out, and everyone cheered.

My mind was spinning. I secretly really wanted at least one girl, but I needed to make peace with myself so I would not be disappointed if the second baby turned out to be a boy. I didn't start contracting again right away and had about forty-five minutes of rest and skin to skin with little baby Bert. Finally, he was taken from me and I was told to start pushing even though I wasn't feeling the urge. My water had broken two days before (I'd been heavily leaking pinkish fluid) and the midwives didn't want to waste another minute. As I began to push, the contractions picked back up, but the intensity was nothing like it had been with the first one. Fifteen minutes later, Baby B was crowning, and with one more push, Baby B was out. This time I was anxious to know the gender immediately, but the cord was short and wrapped around Baby B's little neck. As Pita unwound the cord, I heard whispers of "no pulse." Quickly, I felt under the water, between the baby's legs, and to my utter delight, there was no bulk there. "It's a girl," I cried out. Jennifer cheered, but the midwives were too focused on the still, gray figure to notice my discovery. Pita was rubbing her little body and puffing small breaths into her mouth. "Talk to your baby," she instructed me. "Miriam," I sang, "Little Miri baby, do you hear your mama?" Suddenly she gasped and let out a squawking cry that was music to our ears. I cradled Miriam in my arms and looked around in wonder. I had done it! I had labored through the pain of a separated rib to birth two completely perfect babies: a boy *and* a girl, in the warmly lit comfort of my little house in the country.

After a few more minutes in the water with Miriam, I handed her off and slowly climbed out of the tub. I delivered both placentas on the toilet about forty-five minutes later, and Jennifer whisked them away to be made into powdered capsules, which she would deliver three days later. I showered, put clothes on, and at midnight, my family arrived to meet the babies. We all gathered in our bedroom, and I laid in bed while the midwives looked the babies over, weighing and measuring and swaddling. Someone poured glasses of white wine. Someone fed me almonds and apples. Jennifer left exactly twenty-four hours after she had arrived. The midwives left just eight hours after their arrival. As we all tucked in for the night, I gazed in wonder at the perfect tiny faces snuggled between my husband and I, and snapped a picture of the four of us. When I look at that picture now, I can't help but laugh at how naive I was.

Miracle Baby Bea in Ireland

○ ○ ○ ○ ○ ○ ○ ○ ● ● ○ ○ ○ ● ● ○ ● ○

"Considering my age, forty-two, and having had previous miscarriages, I thought I would never be able to experience a home birth. Thankfully, I found a midwifery team who thought differently."

—Becky, solicitor
Wicklow, Ireland

I was induced with my first daughter, Zoë, in St. Thomas's Hospital in London. My hopes for a water birth using hypnotherapy disappeared very quickly once the drugs to induce me kicked in. I ended up having an epidural and an episiotomy. I was told I was one push away from a C-section owing to Zoë getting distressed at the end of thirty hours of labor. Although delighted by Zoë's safe arrival and also to have escaped a C-section, I never felt reconciled to having my choices in labor taken away and the feeling that I hadn't been listened to.

Midwife-led care in Dublin didn't cover where we live in Wicklow, so when I became pregnant with Bea, I booked into the National Maternity Hospital, Holles Street, for a hospital birth (the home birth service provided through Holles Street, was unlikely to take me on, as I had lost two babies through miscarriage between Zoë and my amazing miracle baby, Bea). I knew they would have classed me as a high-risk pregnancy and not eligible for home birth owing to my age (forty-two), but when I was about five months pregnant with Bea, I realized that I was getting increasingly uneasy about Holles Street's policy on induction and their requirement to be in established labor within twelve hours of the onset of labor; I really only like deadlines if I am the one setting them!

During a conversation with a local midwife, I was told about a home birth service provided by UK Birth Centres (UKBC). I'd flirted with the idea of a home birth with Zoë, but I didn't have the courage as a first-time mom to go for it. I contacted UKBC to see if they covered Wicklow. I also inquired if I was considered to be a low-risk pregnancy that they would take on. Amazingly, they said despite being forty-two and having had previous miscarriages, they considered me a low-risk pregnancy and could take me on, as they had capacity. They suggested a meeting with one of their midwives, Liz, for me and my husband, Kilian, to talk through some of our questions and concerns about home birth. I'm a lawyer and Kilian is a journalist, so the list of questions was very long! After grilling Liz for two hours about the risks of birthing at home and how hospital transfers are managed, both Kilian and I were satisfied that a home birth might actually be less risky than trying to time my journey up to Dublin so that I arrived in Holles Street only once I was in established labor. Having not labored naturally the last time, I didn't know how long it would take me to get into established labor, and I worried about giving birth on the highway! Liz patiently gave us all the facts, was candid about the risks, and very clear about how they were managed. We both felt very reassured after talking to Liz and agreed we would give home birth a go.

Liz started her visits to us at thirty-two weeks, and it was great fun getting to know her. Zoë absolutely loved being present for her visits and watching Liz check the bump and my blood pressure. It was so nice that Zoë could be involved in some of the preparations for the baby.

As I got near to my due date, we realized Bea was lying spine-to-spine. Liz has a sixth sense for knowing what to suggest. She linked the back pain and Symphysis Pubis Dysfunction (SPD) I had been having with my pelvis not being completely straight. She felt this was stopping Bea from getting into the right position and recommended that I see my osteopath to get the issue sorted out. After my first session, Bea turned Right Occiput (ROA). She moved back into spine-to-spine position a week later so we tried some Rozobo work and another osteopath session. Bea then turned Left Occiput Anterior (LOA).

Liz's advice on what to be thinking about was perfectly tuned in with each week of my pregnancy. I never felt overloaded with information, but I had all the evidence-based information I needed at exactly the right stage. As we got nearer to my estimated due date (EDD), Liz talked to me about all my birth preferences and helped me form a birth plan.

Bea was "due" on December 9th, and my plan was to have her on time, get breastfeeding established, and then get my little family over to England to spend Christmas with my folks. Of course, Bea had a different plan, so we sailed past my EDD with no sign of our little miracle baby. I shelved my plans for a Christmas with my folks, and tried very hard to be patient (not an easy task for me). The week after my EDD, Liz had to go to the UK on a day course that was critical for her continued professional indemnity insurance cover. Even though I felt sure I would be unable to go into labor when I knew Liz was not available, Dan (the second midwife—called "the boy midwife" by Zoë) insisted on spending the day in and around Wicklow so that he could be nearby in case I went into labor. He also made a special trip down to Wicklow the week before to meet me so that he could look at my birth plan and make sure I was comfortable with the care being provided.

We got into the second week past my EDD, and I was beginning to fret that I would end up being induced at forty-two weeks pregnant. I booked a placenta scan for the week after Christmas and we tried all manner of things to encourage Bea to make an appearance: curry, hot baths, long walks up hills, Robozo work, homeopathic remedies, as well as talking to Bea. Finally, on the 22nd of December, after a few days with a bit of bleeding and some strong cramps, I woke up to a strong feeling that it was all going to kick off. Zoë had been taken out to spend the day ice skating with some cousins while our au pair was back in Germany visiting her folks for Christmas. All was quiet, nothing was stirring, not even a mouse. At last, I had peace and quiet and space in my nest. I spent the morning making vegetarian sage stuffing from the sage bush in my polytunnel and some Christmas biscuits. I had to keep stopping to breathe through a few erratic contractions. After lunch, Kilian dragged me up the hill behind our house; I was really glad to get out and felt the walking would help keep things happening. By evening I wanted the transcutaneous electrical nerve stimulation (TENS) machine* on, and by 9:30 p.m. I decided I wanted to get in the pool. We kept Liz up to speed with developments all day. Kil called her around 8:30 p.m. to say she might want to come down as it no longer looked like a false alarm!

I was in the birthing pool, in baby's room, and I was enjoying some of my favorite music. At one point, Kilian played me a Manu Chou song; the rhythm of that was just perfect for focusing on breathing and contractions! Although the contractions were getting more frequent, I felt happy that I was where I wanted to be and that we were finally on the road to meeting Bea. Liz arrived about 10:30 p.m. and sat with me while Kil slept for a couple of hours (we knew it would be a long night). By 3:00 a.m. I'd already had three big contractions, and Liz decided I was probably in established labor, so she called Dan. Interestingly, my contractions were never regular so I would never have known when to get in the car to Holles Street if I had still been doing a hospital birth! By the time Dan arrived, I was finding the contractions quite tough. Liz encouraged me to use some gas and air, and Dan took over holding my hand and encouraging me through the toughest bits. I remember being shattered at that point. I really felt I had run out of energy (hardly surprising, as I was missing a night's sleep). Liz started using some of the homeopathic remedies that my homeopathic practitioner (Ashleigh) had provided, and we carried on making progress (albeit slowly).

I was still in the pool, but once I started pushing, it became clear that we had hit a bit of a problem. As with my labor with Zoë, my cervix had become very swollen, so it was going to be very difficult to get Bea out. Liz decided to try ice and a homeopathic remedy, Sepia.** By this point, I

* A TENS machine uses electro stimulation for pain management, back pain, and rehabilitation.
** "*The Family Guide to Homoeopathy*" by Dr. Andrew Lockie explains that Sepia (the source of which is cuttlefish ink) 'is used in conditions characterized by stasis—a state of stoppage in which nervous and hormonal impulses seem to be canceling each other out.' That is a perfect description of where I was at in labor; my poor body was desperately trying to birth my baby, but my fear held me back and produced that big swollen cervix that was slowing me down." —Becky Clissmann

was roaring for an epidural (even though I knew I didn't *really* want one), and a hospital transfer seemed likely. Amazingly the ice/Sepia combination worked, and twenty minutes later, the swelling had stopped completely. Liz said afterward that she had not seen a worse case of edema; the effect of ice alone could not account for the way the swelling reduced. I knew the homeopathic remedies would be key to a good birth!

For some reason that I still can't fathom, and despite having desperately wanted a water birth with both my pregnancies, I decided to leave the pool; I just suddenly knew that my baby would be born on land even though it would be harder for me (I find water really is the best pain management tool in labor). Dan decided to hypnotize me, and as soon as I was relaxed, my waters went. I began pushing in earnest, and after what seemed like a very long time, Bea's head was born. With the next contraction, Liz instantly realized we had another problem: a bilateral shoulder dystocia. These are thankfully quite rare and only occur in about 2 percent of births. Basically, both of Bea's shoulders were wedged in my pelvis. We were into a full-on obstetric emergency. I was only dimly aware of all this. My contractions had stopped, and Liz had to try three different maneuvers before Bea was finally born. This involved all three of them (Dan, Liz, and Kilian) moving me onto all fours, and then onto my back for a McRoberts maneuver—basically the midwife has to twist the baby free. It took three attempts at the McRoberts maneuver before Bea came out. I didn't know it at the time, but Kilian told me that the resuscitation kit was all rolled out on the bed in anticipation of having to revive Bea, but she started screaming as she came out (she's a feisty little thing). Liz told me the next day that Bea was the most amazing pink color when she came out—top of the Apgar score!

The third stage of my labor had to be managed with drugs as I was bleeding quite a bit; post-partum hemorrhage is a risk with shoulder dystocia. However, as Liz and I had discussed, she clamped and cut the cord as high up as possible to allow Bea as much cord blood as possible (approximately 30 percent of a baby's blood is in the placenta and cord during birth to make delivery easier, so cutting the cord too early can cause a baby to lose up to 30 percent of its blood). While Liz worked away to stem the blood flow and deliver the placenta, Bea started feeding. I just remember feeling so content. I was at home, in bed, after delivering my baby—it was one of the happiest moments in my life. Once Liz was happy that I was out of danger, we all had a homeopathic remedy (Aconite IM), a cup of tea, and some toast with local honey, and calmed down before we all had a bit of a nap.

I was very lucky that despite the McRoberts maneuver, I only tore a tiny bit. It was a good clean tear on the line of where I had been stitched after my episiotomy from Zoë's birth, so Liz decided no stitches were needed this time. I think being in the water for so long before Bea was born had softened my skin, making all the stretching possible. A couple of weeks later, and aided by some homeopathic remedies, I was feeling much better-healed than I had after Zoë's birth.

Although the final part of Bea's birth was obviously not what I had hoped for, I am of the view that it was actually safer to have faced that sort of emergency at home. I was in the hands of two experienced midwives that I knew and trusted. A diagnosis was made immediately; I've read that you generally have about five to six minutes to deliver the rest of the baby in this sort of situation or else the outcome can be very poor. Liz knew what I was capable of, and I knew that when Liz issued instructions (as opposed to recommendations or suggestions) that she needed me to comply immediately, without wasting time. The room only had the four of us in it—no useless spectators—just the people who cared about me and who could save my baby. We didn't have to wait for a consultant to answer a call; Liz leapt into action immediately. Also, I hadn't had an epidural (something that I might have succumbed to in hospital) so it was easier for the three of them to move me around to enable the various procedures.

Birth is always an unpredictable journey, but I felt safe in my nest with "the best midwife in the world" (Zoë's name for Liz) with me. Most of my labor was calm and focused and, most importantly, was how I wanted it to be. I feel immensely privileged to have experienced the magic of a natural birth with minimal interventions right from the first cramps to finally holding my wonderful baby skin-on-skin for a good two hours after birth. Given my age and the fact that it was so difficult to get pregnant, it is unlikely that I will be pregnant again. But if I were, I would choose home birth again without hesitation.

Frank Breech Babe

○ ○ ○ ○ ○ ○ ○ ○ ○ ● ○ ○ ○ ○ ○ ○ ● ○

"I feel like many of us grow up knowing little to nothing about birth, so when the time comes, the 'norm' seems to be that you go to a hospital. It's very empowering to know what our bodies and babies are capable of."

—Raychel, mother of four
Vancouver, Washington

As with many birth stories, this one must begin a few days before my baby boy decided to make his way earth-side. I had been experiencing pre-labor contractions for a while at this point, which I tried to convince myself were helping my body prepare for the real thing. I was so done; this was my last baby, and I was ready to hold him in my arms instead of inside my aching body!

Four days before my due date, I made my way to my appointment with my midwives, Mary and Pita. After being palpated multiple times by my midwife, her daughter, and their assistant, along with listening for heart tones, they determined that our baby was likely in a breech position. I was so upset; what would this mean for us? I knew that the local hospitals would not allow for anything other than a Cesarean, but what about my midwives? Mary and Pita were reassuring as we discussed that breech is just another variation of birth positioning, and they were confident in my ability to have this baby. They suggested different techniques I could do to coax him to turn, which I began doing that day. Mary and Pita encouraged me join the Facebook group, Coalition for Breech Birth, so I could read other successful breech birth stories, and I watched a natural breech birth video I found online.

In an effort to gain as much information as possible and to verify his exact position, our midwife ordered an ultrasound for the following day.

Sure enough, my baby was Frank breech: feet up near his face. At this point, I was only three days away from my due date. I was doing inversions, getting chiropractic adjustments, and acupuncture with moxibustion treatments. I opted not to go into the hospital for an external cephalic version (ECV), because I was nervous about the potential risks. I was especially confident with not going to the hospital knowing that I had a skilled birth team who would help me deliver him regardless of his position.

When I learned that Silas was Frank breech, I was fearful in the sense that I had never had a breech birth before, and I had no way of knowing how it would affect my labor. Between consulting with my experienced midwives and conducting my own research, I didn't see a breech birth as being an emergency, and we decided to continue with the home birth while hoping that Silas would turn head-down.

On August 22nd, my estimated due date, things started picking up and becoming slightly more uncomfortable. My friend and doula, Ann, came over to help me and ended up driving me to an acupuncture appointment. Another friend and birth photographer, Karyn, joined us later in case things progressed; sadly, they didn't. I sent my friends home and climbed into bed to get some rest. Little did I know, things were about to pick up soon!

I was able to sleep most of the night, but in the early morning of August 23rd, I started having difficulty sleeping through my contractions. I still questioned if this was "the real deal," but I texted Pita at 7:45 a.m. when contractions were two to four minutes apart, and when I needed to breathe through them. She asked a few questions and told me she would get things ready and come check on me soon. I told her there was no need to rush and that most of my family was still sleeping.

I texted her again at about 9:15 a.m. to let her know that my other three kids and husband were now awake and that things were getting a bit more painful, to which she responded that she was on her way. I also texted my doula and photographer to let them know we were getting close.

When Pita arrived at my house, she checked me for dilation at my request and I was at a three. I let Ann and Karyn know so they could head over. I continued to labor in my bed while my husband, Joel, and Pita started getting my birth tub ready. After some time had passed, I decided I wanted to get into the now-ready birth tub. Pita checked me again to see if I had progressed, and I was now at five centimeters dilated. The warm water helped to relax my muscles. My friends arrived shortly after, along with my other midwife and their assistant.

My daughters, Mirka and Stella, asked if they could come in the "birth bath" for a bit, and I welcomed them in. My eldest, Ezekiel, was happy to play his computer game for most of my labor as he's "been there, done that" with seeing Stella's birth! I continued to labor for quite a while in the tub, now supported by my husband and entire birth team. I asked to be checked once again, only to find out I was still at five centimeters. I felt a bit discouraged as I had not experienced a long labor with my other three births, and we were already ten hours in at this point!

My team convinced me to get out and labor standing up to allow movement and gravity to help things along. I did this for a while and then suddenly started becoming very emotional and crying. I began to feel ill and ran for the bathroom where I threw up and continued crying.

Part of me thought, *could this be transition?*

That must have been what everyone else thought too, because they suggested we make our way to the bed for another check. Still at five centimeters! What the heck? I had been stuck at five centimeters for five hours!

At this point, Mary and Pita thought it best to call a doctor they knew at the hospital to see about driving me in for an ultrasound. They said it was possible there was a reason Silas wasn't engaging. I became very upset and nervous because I was convinced if I showed up at the hospital, very obviously in labor with a breech baby, they would not let me leave. Of course, if there was a real danger to myself or the baby, I wouldn't be against staying at the hospital, but I wasn't aware of anything being wrong at this point beyond the slow progression.

Everyone other than my husband left the room to leave us alone while Mary made the call. I started quietly, yet firmly telling Silas that we were going to have to go to the hospital if he didn't come right now and to please, please come down. I stood up and had two or three contractions in the ten minutes that I was standing up against the wall and all of the sudden, I felt like something was coming out! I yelled at Joel that something was coming out, who then yelled for the midwives to come. Pita got there first and quickly checked me while I was still standing. I went from five centimeters to ten centimeters in that span of ten minutes we were alone in the room!! She told me that I was complete and his bum was right there!

The birth team worked quickly to put down my waterproof birth blanket on our bed and helped me onto it. My water broke with the first contraction on the bed. They stacked pillows for me to lean over while I was on my hands and knees, but I kept sinking into them. Joel laid down on the pillows and I leaned on top of his back for stability. Mary and Pita told me not to push until I absolutely couldn't refrain, and I tried my best to follow their advice. After a couple of minutes, I just had to begin pushing! Things moved very quickly. In fact, Silas became very impatient to be born; it took only two minutes and twenty-eight seconds from when his bum started to crown until he was fully delivered! Later, I learned from the photos that Karyn took, Silas wanted to be here so badly that he pulled his own legs and arms out by himself, one at a time. It was my longest labor at almost twelve hours, and it was certainly the most different! Silas was eight pounds fourteen ounces twenty-one and a half inches long, and was born at 5:07 p.m. on August 23rd, 2015.

Chapter 4

You Gave Birth Where?

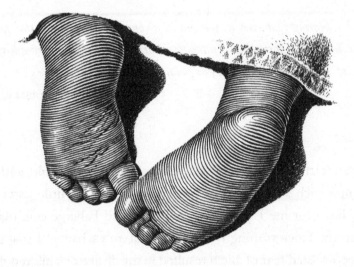

Oren's Birth in a Converted Cow Shed in Ireland

○ ○ ○ ○ ○ ○ ○ ○ ○ ○ ○ ○ ○ ○ ○ ○ ‹ ○

"I remember hearing that even if you are in a coma, your body will still give birth. That information transformed me. In this moment, I am effortlessly surrendering to the experience of birth, and it's not scary or painful."

—Kathryn, social ecologist
Ireland

I have been terrified of birth my whole life. When I was a child, and before I even knew such a thing was possible, I would tell my little sister that if she gave birth for me I would buy her a jeweled Fabergé egg; that must have been the fanciest thing I could think of to exchange! I suspect that such a deep-rooted fear of birth resulted in my dislike of children through my teens and twenties and my determination to be permanently child-free well into my thirties.

When I found out I was pregnant, I immediately realized just how much fear I had about birth and parenting. Despite being in a stable, fulfilling relationship for two years with a man I'd loved for sixteen years, I knew then that my indecision about whether to have kids would have remained until I no longer had a choice; time would have made it for me. As the months passed, I unpacked layer after layer of my stuff, my mother's stuff, her mother's stuff, and a whole load of society's stuff. All this "stuff" revolved around being pregnant, giving birth, being a parent, and discovering my own identity. I dived in with both feet, as is my tendency, and explored each fear as it arose.

Birth was going to be painful, traumatizing, and utterly horrific. I had no idea how I would get through it. I knew there were plenty of health benefits for me and baby to have a natural, drug-free birth, so I started researching how to achieve that. I was upset to find that most women in hospitals do not have the birth they hope for. When I dug further, it seemed that hospitals often cause difficult and painful births with their bright lights, busy wards, and policies of managing labor along strict time lines. One simple intervention can lead to another, and before you know it, you are having an episiotomy or C-section. Some hospitals in Ireland have a 40 percent C-section rate and an 80 percent episiotomy rate—way beyond what should be needed according to the World Health Organization.

I began seeking alternatives and discovered that home births are shown to be just as safe and often with happier outcomes than hospital births. Hurray! I felt so much hope. I thought I could just call up my local home birth midwife and book one. I was outraged to be told that Ireland's Health Service Executive (HSE) does not provide enough support for the 10 percent of women who request a home birth midwife; as a result, only 1 percent of women are granted a home birth. There just aren't enough midwives to go around, and the HSE rules keep making it harder and harder for midwives to do their jobs. I phoned all eighteen midwives on the list until luck was eventually on my side. I found a midwife available for my due date in October, but home birth guidelines in Ireland require midwives to be two hours from the client's place of birth; our home was more than the two hours away from the midwife available to us. Thankfully, my friend who lived near our midwife was going to be away, and offered us her home for the birth. Our midwife did all my prenatal checks at home; no hospital queues for me, except for a single scan.

The other tool I found was called HypnoBirthing; a course that educated me about the physiology of birth, and helped me understand everything that would happen in my body during labor. It also gave me a practice for staying relaxed during labor and a whole range of techniques for reducing fear, pain, and worry during pregnancy and birth. I never deeply believed it would work, but as it was the only technique I had, I decided to allow myself to pretend a little and believe it would give me the "comfortable, easy birth" it said it would.

Just four weeks before my due date, the home my friend offered us to birth in was no longer available. Panic stations! We had to find another place within our midwife's area. A stressful two weeks of research and calls ensued until I found a place on Airbnb that I instantly knew was right. It was called Fairy Fort Farm, and the owner's picture captured a salt-of-the-earth kinda guy; I liked him instantly. I typed yet another "no room at the inn" email. He responded with warmth, excitement, and a resounding yes that the stable, converted into a cottage, was available! I could not make this stuff up. He would love a baby born on the farm, the first in one hundred years! We were heading to Tipperary. We decided to book the whole month, not knowing when I would deliver exactly, with my estimated due date being October 12th.

October 3rd was moving day. I had a scary show of a little blood the night before, but a text to my midwife put me at ease; with no other symptoms, I could still be weeks away from going into labor. I was weepy and emotional to be packing up and leaving my folks and everyone I knew. I took in that the next time I'd be home, everything would be different and, if all went well, we would have a baby! It was scary, and I felt mopey and had a bath instead of getting on the road in the early morning like we should have.

My mum drove Jordan and I down after lunch. About an hour and a half into the trip I realized I was having super mild contractions. They were no big deal, so I didn't mention them. I stretched my body out as flat as I could in the passenger seat and breathed. After a couple more contractions, Jordan realized what was happening and decided to time them. I reassured him that there was nothing happening and not to bother. After a few more contractions in quick succession, Jordan timed them anyway; they were 3 minutes apart. I laughed and said, "It's just the emotions of the move." I believed it, too, as the Braxton Hicks sessions I'd had on and off for the past three months had all been way more intense.

We stopped off on the way to pick up supplies. I felt subdued as I walk in the rain down Westport main street managing mild, mostly annoying, but barely present contractions. Mum and Jordan commented on how miserable I looked. I'm not sure that I was miserable, but I definitely wasn't happy.

I was actively managing the contractions when we arrived at the farm. It took a little energy and effort to focus, breathe, and stay calm. As we drove up the little country lane, a cockerel began walking slowly in front of the car, right down the grassy line in the middle of the lane. Turning his head from side to side, he looked like a proud welcoming representative. We laughed, and I started feeling excited to be in such a magical place. When we entered the courtyard of the farm buildings, Michael was there, smiling and happy at our arrival. He had a farm volunteer with him, and I got a sudden surge of panic that he had put her in the same cottage as us. I feared I made a big mistake, and that I wouldn't be getting the privacy I needed. My stressed state escalated gradually. In the bedroom, I became even more upset, panicking that this was a stupid idea while also fretting that there was no lunch and no dinner, and thinking that maybe these contractions did mean something. They were getting quite intense. Actually, they were painful. I didn't think I could do this . . . and I needed to poo. Yes. I read that some women need to empty their bowels before labor begins. That must be what this was. I had a strong urge to . . . poo. I was a little frantic in energy now. Jordan and Mum tried to assure me that they would unpack and have food ready, and that I should just go lie down, listen to my HypnoBirthing tracks, and relax. I tried, but I couldn't. *I needed to poo.*

I went to the toilet; nothing happened but a rising stress level and a need to push out a poo. I tried again to relax. Nothing. I jumped up. Trying to stay calm, I said, "This is bullshit. What was I thinking having a home birth? In the middle of nowhere? I can't do this. I am going to end up in hospital with a C-section."

Mum replied, "You won't. I know you can do this; that will not happen to you!"

I believed her. Jordan was being loving and supportive and desperately trying to get me in the hypno-zone. It wasn't working. I headed back to the toilet.

"Are you pushing, Kat?" He shouted through the bathroom door.

"No! I need to poo, okay? Give me some privacy!" I shouted.

Jordan shouted back, "You're pushing! Stop it, it's way too early! You'll do damage!"

He came in and tried to get me to come outside for a walk with him. I reluctantly allowed myself to be led until we got to the door, and I suddenly, yet firmly said, "No, I am not going. I need Helen! Call Helen. I need support. I can't do this! She said she would be there for support if I freaked. I am freaking. Call her." I headed back to the bathroom to follow my urge to poo. I was gripping the towel rail which was mounted strongly into the old stone wall. I was pulling it with all my might. Pushing. I listened through the door as Jordan, in his typical, calm way, called Helen and told her I was asking for her support. She said she would be right there.

I felt an immediate sense of calm and headed to the bed with Jordan's encouragement. He put on the HypnoBirthing tracks, and I easily got in the zone. I felt in control and content, but in a slightly altered state. Everything was kind of hazy and zoned out. I had several more contractions, and I felt calm, centered, and totally in control of the experience. This was good. I felt relaxed, and there was no pain, just the gentle rising and falling of my uterus as it tightened its muscles.

Helen entered the room like a gentle breeze: no drama, just sweet and gentle understanding.

"What's going on, Kathryn?" She breathed in the calmest, most supportive of tones.

"Oh Helen, I'm just so afraid you're going to tell me I am not even in labor proper, and this is already so intense, and I am afraid I can't do this."

"Okay, what do you need?"

"I need an internal exam to tell me what is happening."

I barely noticed the procedure, it was so unobtrusive. Helen looked at me, and I could see subtle surprise on her face.

"What's your best-case scenario, Kathryn?"

I thought to myself, that is a really mean question to ask a woman in labor! But I responded truthfully, "Ten centimeters and ready to push."

"You're ten centimeters and ready to push. Actually, the baby is already two centimeters out of the cervix."

Wait . . . what?

"You're some woman! How did you do that, Kathryn?"

I have no idea how I did that.

Helen said she must call the second midwife and the hospital as procedure. She told me to keep doing what I was doing. I felt absolutely no concern. I trusted that birth was natural and my body was doing what it needed to do. I remember hearing that even if you are in a coma, your body will still give birth. That information transformed me. I was effortlessly surrendering to the experience, and it wasn't scary or painful. In fact, if I allowed myself to be honest, I was enjoying it. Not in an "orgasmic birth" kind of way (yes, they exist!), but more in a wow, look what I am feeling, I can sense *everything* kind of way. I could feel the movements of my body slowly and gently moving a baby down. It was all so interesting. I realized this must be what I had read about; that the body will continue to open and the baby will move down effortlessly and painlessly.

I had been so afraid that I was not "embodied enough" to have a natural, pain-free birth. That my over-analytic mind would get in the way, and I wouldn't be able to surrender like the books said I should. And yet, what actually happened was that I used all my mental capacity to help me connect more deeply with what was going on in my body. My mind and body worked as one in the most embodied way I could ever have imagined. I felt so elated and liberated at this realization . . . like I was not broken or too in my head. I have an inquisitive mind and was able to find a way to use that knowledge to access my own bodily wisdom . . . or something like that.

So, I was ten centimeters and ready to push! Mum came running in from the other room where she had been praying. She was elated and loud and congratulatory exclaiming, "You did it! You did it! I knew you could!" I was happy, but I was trying to stay calm and in the zone so I could tell her that, and she tried to calm herself a little. I was aware of how lovely this was. I had only done part of the labor, but it was wonderful to have her here (she was meant to drop us off and leave), being typically supportive.

I continued lying there and breathing for a while. I don't know how long, maybe an hour. At some point, I followed the urge to change positions regularly and effortlessly.

Jordan, who had been in and out of the room trying to make dinner, unpack the car, fill the pool, and prepare lunch, was now with me completely.

I required constant pressure on my lower back, and I regularly shouted, "*More Pressure!*" Jordan is strong, so I couldn't understand why he was pushing so lightly. I was frequently up on my knees. I began to feel hot in the body and called out for something cool. The next sensation was a shock: a wet, cold, heavy material had been thrown across my back. I think I screamed and probably cursed. It was the second midwife, and I was annoyed that she didn't give me warning. It felt like an eternity between request and delivery, yet it was probably moments.

Time was hazy as I frequently leapt about the bed to change positions and made demands (chocolate, water, pressure, coldness, dimness), until I decided I was probably tired and should lie down.

I lay on my back; Helen said I shouldn't. She emphasized that it's the worst position for labor, but I thought I would just take a minute to rest here. The discomfort and intolerance of the position was almost instant, so I leapt up again. No wonder hospital births are often experienced as difficult!

I lay on my side resting. It seemed like things had grown quieter inside, and I was not feeling the uncontrollable urges to push.

Helen said "Just keep following the urges to push."

I told her they weren't really there anymore.

She said, "Give me your hand."

She placed my hand down where I could feel the bulge of the sac of unbroken waters! It was kind of gross and intense. As much as I would love to be one of those "wow, that's so beautiful" type of women, I'm more "ugh, that's full-on."

She asked me if I wanted to look with a mirror, and I shrieked with half a laugh, "No!"

She said we were getting close. I asked her why things seemed to have slowed down. Our midwife knew I needed to understand things biologically and emotionally.

So, she plainly stated, "Well, some women have a little fear when it comes to the pushing out stage."

That seemed to me to be true, and I nodded. The second midwife asked if I wanted some herbal support and then held a bottle of Clarry Sage under my nose. *Boom.* The contractions and urge to push hit as hard as a high, and we were off again. I remember making a deep, loud note. It was operatic, and I held it for what seemed like a long, beautiful moment.

At some stage shortly after, I caught a whiff of nervousness from the midwives. It was almost imperceptible and well-covered, but I caught it nonetheless. I was still hyperaware of my surroundings when I needed to be, despite this altered state.

I think they had just done a check on me, and Helen said, "Okay, let's move this on more quickly. I want you to do a couple of big pushes to get this baby out."

I was really quite taken aback. I was assured that there would be no coached pushing in a home birth. No midwives or doctors shouting "push," because there was simply no need in a natural, physiological birth. And yet they seemed to be telling me to push. I had been doing the HypnoBirthing "breathing down" technique; a very gentle breathing that nudges the baby down little by little with each contraction. I was loving the ease and trust it was generating in me. But now things were moving faster, my stress started to build.

Helen said, "Okay, Kathryn, take a big breath and push down hard!"

Wait . . . what? How? Like this?

No.

Okay . . . like this?

Jordan said, "No, close your mouth and push instead of breath. Push down hard with your mouth closed. With all your might."

Helen interjected, "We only need two of these . . . I can see baby's head . . . just two big pushes and the baby will be out!"

She tells me she is going to break the waters, and I want to argue, but don't.

I tried to push another time, but I was feeling pissed off that this was happening so fast. I picked up on the urgency again and took it seriously.

Push.

Okay. It felt intense but not painful. I could feel a stretching and a burning. I knew this was called the ring of fire, it is common, and it means birth is imminent. It was not taking a lot of energy to do this. I was pushing with maybe 50 percent of my capacity. I called for my mum so she could witness the birth, and she ran in.

Helen said, "One more push, Kathryn, a big one."

I pushed again with maybe 70 percent. I know I was afraid. I was afraid of something being wrong, of pain starting now, of tearing, and of all this beautiful birthing being over and of parenting beginning.

But there was no choice now, no time for anything else. I pushed and whooshed and, no slop, I looked beneath and baby was not on the bed. Our baby was in midair! Arms reached out and suddenly there was a baby boy lying as clean as a whistle on the bed. I went into self-care mode. Again, I wish I was one of those women who went straight into gushing, looking, and watching; but I didn't. I was a little overwhelmed by the physicality of what I just did. I was not in "parent mode" as most birth videos show. Instead, I was in *am I okay?* mode, *aren't I amazing for doing all that?* mode. I looked to connect with Jordan, but he was peering excitedly past me to the baby. We had a brief moment to exchange looks, and he jumped up and went to the baby. Things were happening with the baby. An oxygen mask gave a single breath of air. Things were calm though, and there didn't seem to be any need to worry. They all took the baby to the other room, just beyond the door of this two room converted cow shed we were renting. I could see them all in the half-light; smiling and excited and laughing. Helen was weighing him in a little white cloth, tied like in the cartoons of a stork delivery, and calling out the time of birth. It was 9:20 p.m., only four hours since our arrival at the cottage, and five and a half since labor began in the car.

I lay back on the bed, watching from a distance, feeling a little left out and excluded from the celebration. The second midwife, Brenda, told me we should deliver the placenta now. Shit! I had forgotten about that! I lamented, "That's like a whole other delivery, isn't it? Oh no! It's not over after all."

"No," she said, "just kneel up on the bed there."

She put a bowl beneath me, and with a plop, the placenta simply dropped out. I couldn't believe the ease, and I laughed with the relief of it.

Helen came back in and said she needed to check me for tears, as it was best to do stitches while the birth hormones are still high to reduce the pain. She was swift and gentle and immediately told me I didn't have a scratch! I was so, so pleased. My big fear was tearing, stitches, and un-bearable pain. I was now through the whole thing, and none of those things happened! There were no words for the relief and pride in my preparation and accomplishment. I felt big. I felt strong. I felt capable. I did it! I had a baby at home with no pain, no tears, no drugs. I was celebrating myself and am not really connecting to the reality of having a baby.

The baby was brought back into the room, and I was told I should breastfeed. It felt rushed and forced on me. I had no time to really look at my baby, to see him, to connect; I must latch him on!

Breastfeeding was a whole other thing. I had never done this either and had no idea what to do. Helen lifted him onto me and I think I was in shock at the reality of having an actual baby. I had been so focused on getting through the birth unscathed that I really hadn't expected that there would be a baby at the end. And now here he was. I know I was meant to feel gushy and overwhelmed, but I didn't. I felt shocked and surprised and a bit invaded. I was so busy congratulating myself that I forgot there was more work to be done!

Everyone else's joy and excitement made me overwhelmingly invisible, about which I felt glad. I got on with the task of trying to get the latch right. Trying to hold the baby gently. Trying to know what to feel. Trying to feel free to feel what I am feeling.

I looked at the baby. He was so tiny, so perfect, and so utterly focused on me. His eyes were open, and he was looking at me. He was beautiful with dark hair and a lovely color to his skin. His tiny hands grasped, and he seemed to know what to do about feeding. Time slips away . . . vague memories of phone calls being made, photos being taken, midwives leaving advice for the night, food, bed, fire, hugs, excitement, joy, looking, watching, fear, confidence. Jordan's support and love, my mum's ecstasy. And a baby.

On a Barge in Ireland

○ ○ ○ ○ ○ ○ ○ ○ • • ○ • ○ • ○ ○ (○

"While we were all on the tiny bed, during two surges, we heard a knock on the hull. We all turned to look and wondered what it was. I suggested the barge was hitting the jetty, but Neil said the ropes were tight. We thought no more of it as my surges continued. That first night, as I was feeding Finn I heard the knocking again, several times, followed by splashing. I have heard of the otters knocking on hulls in other remote parts of the canal, but never here in the docks. I haven't heard them since; they were Finn's little welcoming party."

—Eibhlín, teacher
Dublin, Ireland

After a couple weeks of twinges, excitement, impatience, and a due date spent in the hairdressers and sipping hot chocolate, at forty weeks and five days, I finally felt a pop followed by a second pop. I was lying in bed at 1:00 a.m., having not slept yet, when I felt my contractions start. I coolly climbed out of bed and made my way to the bathroom where my waters broke—all clear. I made some bread and cheese and called the hospital. I was on the Holles Street Domino home birth scheme which requires a check on vitals for baby and mother when labor begins. I was told to come on in. I woke my husband who, in the confusion, started calling work to tell them he wouldn't make it in. He thought he had gotten a full night's sleep and that it was already morning: the poor guy was in for a surprise.

I was adamant that I was going to walk the ten-minute stroll to the hospital. Just before leaving at around 1:30 a.m., I felt my first surge; it was intense. Stubborn as ever, I continued on with regular surges only a few minutes apart. I made it halfway to the hospital and gave in. The lovely taxi driver refused to charge us with the condition that we did not name the baby after him! In the waiting room, Neil timed the surges which were two to three minutes apart.

The midwife checked my waters and the baby's heartbeat: all was well. We took a taxi back to the barge without any argument from me. On reaching the barge, I started pacing using the TENS machine and breathing techniques. The barge is forty feet by ten feet. It was tight, but we feel so at home in the barge that I didn't notice it being cramped in any way. I was happy to be somewhere familiar, safe, and comfortable. I squatted and used the yoga ball through some surges, as well. We had a pool (the smallest one I could find) wedged between the stove and the edge of the kitchen units, but we were afraid to start filling it too soon. I spent about an hour in the shower, which felt great and then not great at all. The midwife at the hospital was due to finish her shift at seven thirty and told me to call at seven and let her know how I was getting on. Neil called her at about 5:30 a.m. After a brief chat with me on the phone, she came out to the barge. Neil had just started to fill the pool. When she arrived, I was sitting on the bed with Neil's hoody on, hood up, focused entirely on breathing and with the TENS machine on. Her first comment was, "You are in the throes of it now." She was so encouraging and told me I was dilated six centimeters. At this stage I was obsessed with the pool and kept asking poor Neil when it would be ready. For my husband, filling the pool was the hardest part. We had rented an industrial Burco water boiler, he had the geezer on full blast, and had a hose connected to a tap outside. He was my hero!

When the second midwife arrived, I was eight centimeters. I got into the pool, and it was lovely. I didn't relax for long. Our midwife encouraged me into a position that intensified the surges. I was getting closer to my baby. The midwives were extremely positive and encouraging; they didn't just tell me that I could birth our baby; they insisted that I state it. I was in and out of the pool two or three times, always in a new position. After a very short time, I was told I was dilated ten centimeters and baby was coming.

In jest, the two midwives and I decided the baby was a girl. Neil, to be argumentative, declared our baby was a boy. I was encouraged into pushing positions, but nothing happened; Baby was not budging. I tried lunges on all fours, kneeling. The midwife suggested lying on the bed. She said they usually don't encourage lying down, but I was happy to try.

At this stage, I was exhausted. Neil supported me from behind: all four of us somehow fitting on the tiny bed on the barge. Suddenly, things started happening. One of the midwives brought in some clary sage oil on a tissue. She rubbed my feet and spoke encouragingly to me between surges. Slowly, slowly, slowly, my baby was coming. The midwives said that she was probably very small and had lots of room, so she was slipping back a little each time she moved down the birth canal. Ever so slowly she came down, and I could feel her crown.

As we neared the end, the midwife said, "You're going to squat now."

I thought I couldn't, but somehow, I did just as they said. I trusted every encouraging word they spoke to me. Supported by Neil, four hours after I was fully dilated, our baby was born. My first words were about how beautiful my baby was.

Neils's were, "It's a boy!"

And a boy it was; a big boy! He was nine pounds, thirteen ounces. I held him on my chest, sitting on our bedroom floor and he looked straight into my eyes. The midwife said he was a warrior. I said to Neil that Finn was a warrior. He was delighted, as he had put Finn on our list of boy names. It was settled. I was holding our not so little warrior, Finn.

The midwives saw to me and made sure Finn latched on and that I was comfortable and mobile before leaving. I was delighted and confident knowing they would return in the morning. In fact, the midwives visited eight times after the birth of Finn. Neil, baby Finn and I spent our first day and night on the barge snuggled up in our own bed. It was an incredible experience that neither Neil nor I will ever forget.

If You Can't Birth at Home in Bama, Go to Tennessee

○ ○ ○ ○ ○ ○ ○ ○ ○ ● ○ ○ ○ ○ ○ ○ ● ○

"Traveling across state lines to birth our baby safely involved months of coordination with co-care from an incredible physician in Alabama just in case complications were to arise. It involved drives to Tennessee alone with my other two young children. It involved added stress on my family because of my history of quick deliveries. I mean who wants to have a minivan baby?"

—Jessica, registered nurse
Florence, Alabama

The birth situation in Alabama is a bit tricky and can be confusing, especially if you want options in how you birth your babies. I am a registered nurse, and my husband is a family physician, M.D. We have more than fourteen years of post-high school education in our house. And yet, despite research showing what we found to be true (the midwifery model of care reduces the rate of preterm birth), we were not able to legally choose to have our baby with a midwife of any kind in or outside of a hospital in the state of Alabama. Certified Professional Midwives (CPMs) are currently not recognized anywhere in the state of Alabama, and there is not a licensing protocol for CPMs in Alabama.

As a matter of fact, in a legal manner of speaking, only one type of midwife is acknowledged in the Alabama Code: a Certified Nurse Midwife (CNM). CNMs are legal, but they are underutilized, and the nearest one was more than three hours away at the time we were expecting our third child. As a result of the lack of CNMs in Alabama, my third daughter has a Tennessee birth certificate, and it makes me sad.

My oldest daughter was born at thirty-five weeks and two days. My middle at thirty-seven and one day. My youngest at thirty-eight and two days. Those with a history of preterm birth tend to be at risk for it again. Fortunately, I seem to be trending the opposite direction, but I believe that my family physician, OB, and my Certified Professional Midwife are to thank for that. The midwifery model of care promotes physiologic birth that is not tampered with.

Tennessee licenses their Certified Professional Midwives, regulates them, and has a board to whom we can file a complaint and request peer review for accountability if there is an issue or negligence. Tennessee doesn't prosecute for "practicing nurse midwifery without a license." Also, in Tennessee, my midwife can legally bring level 1 hospital equipment to my home or rented home and be there to assist in case of an emergency while I deliver my child. That midwife is trained in how to stabilize an infant, detect heart murmurs, care for a newborn up to six weeks, manage an emergent hemorrhagic event or an unexpected dystocia, etc. Midwives in Tennessee have relationships with Tennessee doctors because those doctors know that CPMs are legal. In Alabama, it is very difficult to find a competent and caring physician that is also willing to work with a CPM or a client choosing out-of-hospital birth that plans to use a CPM. I consider myself blessed to have found such a thing. I know more than one woman who was dropped from the care of her provider for this reason alone.

People have asked, "Why didn't you just use a CNM in the hospital?"

I wanted to, but the only nearby hospital that had a CNM denied privileges to the new CNM that replaced a retiree. The hospital also forbade the use of hydrotherapy in labor despite my physician's approval. I birthed my oldest daughters on bedside commodes because they didn't have appropriate birth stools or alternative delivery options other than that awful breakaway bed. I am an educated woman, and I would like to be given options with informed consent that allow for certain levels of dignity to be maintained during the work of bringing my precious children into this world.

The choice for us was clear: we would make the forty-five-minute trip to Tennessee for the birth of our third baby with a Certified Professional Midwife. The most challenging part of this choice was finding a friend willing to let me use their home in Tennessee. Thankfully, I was able to find a place to deliver my third daughter. However, we are currently expecting our fourth child as I write this, and still trying to iron out plans. The best option I have at the moment is to call the news station when we hit the road and let them catch the story of a nurse and physician having their baby on the side of the road trying to leave the state for access to safe care.

Back to our third birth story: it was October 7th, and it was pumpkin-picking time. The smell of fall was in the air, and the weather was fairly mild considering the season. I was thirty-eight weeks and two days pregnant and about as ripe as the pumpkins. I noticed some pressure, but never any pain during the day, so I notified the midwife.

She said, "Please just come up here and let me check to make sure you aren't progressing." It's a good thing she strongly suggested we make the trip! I was six centimeters dilated. After the appointment, I went back to Alabama, finished picking pumpkins, and returned for another check only to find that I was almost eight centimeters. I then drove home, arranged childcare for my other two kids, made a trip to Walmart, and drove back on up there to my friend's home around nine that evening. After talking a bit and taking vitals, I received antibiotics for Group B Strep infection (GBS) and then proceeded to have a baby. At 12:37 a.m. on October 8th, my newest pumpkin, Lura, gently entered this world in a cattle trough full of warm water with a sterile liner. Yep, it was a redneck birthing tub! During my birth, I had one woman rubbing my back, my husband holding a cool rag on my head, and another woman checking baby with a Doppler intermittently. I was as close to relaxed as I could be during something aptly referred to as "labor." By 3:00 a.m. I was able to head home, and my midwife came to check on me the very next day. Three hundred pumpkins and a full day of fun with the family later, we had a new knowledge base, a new experience in our life, and a precious little chunk of a baby girl that almost weighed eight pounds!

This was my first out-of-hospital birth, my first experience with a Certified Professional Midwife, and my first real reason to feel frustrated by the missing levels of care in my home state (Alabama). The experience left me thankful to live near the state line, and I was impressed by such a different model of care. I want all women to have access to quality information and access to choices concerning their births. Our own home birth spurred my husband and I to found Safer Birth in Bama (SBB). SBB is a 501(c)3 organization dedicated to educating Alabama citizens about our current state of maternity care and increasing access to care in order to improve outcomes. We host screenings, raise funds, and provide scholarships. Our state ranks forty-ninth in infant mortality, but number one in football . . . something's gotta give.

Chapter 5

Birth Teams of Every Kind

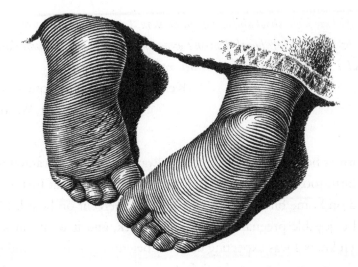

A Young Woman
and Her Little Man

○ ○ ○ ○ ○ ○ ○ ○ ○ ○ ○ ○ ○ ○ ○ ○ ○ ○ ○

"As I grasped my high school diploma at graduation, I never imagined I would be nearly four months pregnant. Although I wasn't expecting to have a baby immediately after high school, I was excited to take on the new role of being a mom."

—Kelsey, stay-at-home mom and nanny
Vancouver, Washington

I was born at home, and I just kind of always knew that I wanted to have a home birth too. My boyfriend, Ben, was a little nervous at first, but once I decided on home birth, he was one hundred percent on board. I had an easy and enjoyable pregnancy; I was never sick, and it went quickly, as I didn't even know I was expecting until the beginning of my second trimester! Good thing, too, because I was forty-two weeks pregnant when I finally started to feel the first contractions on a Wednesday morning.

The contractions were about fifty to twenty minutes apart, but strong enough to wake me up and keep my attention. I came downstairs, turned on the fire, and talked with my dad for a bit. He didn't know I was in labor, and I wanted to keep it that way. The fire felt good, and I kept an eye on my stopwatch. I took natural childbirth classes and had a good idea of what to expect. I wanted to try and be well rested and energized for the labor I knew was about to begin, but it was so hard to not share my excitement!

Around noon the contractions started to become closer together. I stayed home and labored with my mom nearby. My mom suggested we go to one of our favorite stores to walk and get a change of scenery. So, off to Home Depot we went! We walked for about forty minutes before it became too intense. Once home, my dad set up the birthing tub in my parents' room so we would be prepared. Having that detail settled, I had every intention of getting some sleep, but I found myself downstairs in front of the fire once more. The heat was easing some of the pain, and I decided to stay put all night with the warmth. Thankfully, my mom came downstairs and stayed up with me all night.

The next morning, my midwife, Mary, came over to check on my progress and to see how I was doing. I was tired. Very tired. I spent most of the day in the tub; however, I did try moving around to ease some of the pain. I bounced on a yoga ball with a TENS machine on my back, I walked our stairs, and I sat backward on the toilet. Three women from our church came to help with the birth, as well. They were like my third hand. They continually helped me change positions, fed me, got me water, and helped me to the bathroom. I was surrounded by women who only wanted to support me and my birth. It was amazing.

Finally, my midwife basically forced me to get in my parents' bed and try to rest. Trying to rest between rapid contractions was tough. But I hadn't slept in almost two nights. I was exhausted and ready to have our baby in my arms. My parents' bed is adjustable at the head and feet. I was able to elevate myself so I could rest without laying down! It was awesome.

Around 8:45 p.m. on Thursday, Pita asked me if I wanted her to break my water. I agreed. Like I said, I was very tired. I had no sense of time and felt in a complete daze. I also trusted my midwife team completely and agreed that it was the right choice. When my water was broken, there was meconium present. The meconium in my waters wasn't an immediate concern, but something to note and keep an eye on. Baby Owen wasn't showing any signs of distress, and labor was progressing, albeit slowly! For the next four hours, I halfway rested on my parents' bed at nine centimeters dilated; I was so close!

At 12:43 a.m., I was finally complete and pushing! The water in the birth tub had long ago gone cold. Luckily for me, my parents have a great big soaker tub. One of the ladies from our church rolled up some towels for my neck, and the tub was magically filled with perfectly warm water. It felt amazing. During this time my second midwife, Pita, kept me focused. Her calming voice and clear directions were exactly what I needed. I joke that she gave me "the death stare" during the time I was in the tub, but her eye contact kept me in the moment and focused on what I needed to do to have this baby. I had my knees to my chest with my eyes closed just listening to every word Pita said. At one point I was pushing even though I wasn't having a contraction. Pita firmly, yet calmly, told me to push only when I was having a contraction. She kept saying positive notes that kept me looking forward, one contraction at a time. Pita kept her hand on the top of Owen's head as we made our way to crowning. It seemed as though he was stuck in the birth canal for a long time. I finally felt a strong burning sensation and Owen's head crowned, it took another ten minutes of really intense pushing to get the rest of his body out. Owen was born at 2:26 a.m. in my parents' tub, surrounded with love.

Owen was placed on my chest and I exclaimed, "I did it! He's here!" I looked down at Owen and said, "Good job, Buddy." I felt amazing. Fifteen or twenty minutes later the placenta was delivered, and Ben cut the cord. Ben had skin-to-skin with Owen while I showered and dressed.

Although Owen's home birth was amazing, we did encounter a difficult week following his birth. It took a few minutes to get Owen to cry. He came out choking, from what we thought was meconium that got in his lungs. His breathing was heavy, but we were all keeping a close eye. Before my midwives left, around 5:00 a.m., they told me to keep them informed later that morning if Owen's breathing had improved or not. As I laid in my parents' bed, newborn on my chest, I finally squeezed in three hours of sleep. I woke up at 8:00 a.m., texted Mary to tell her that Owen was still breathing pretty heavily, and I wasn't having any luck getting him to nurse. She told me to immediately take him to the emergency room.

Without any further ado, my mom, Ben, and I drove to the hospital. By 10:00 a.m. Owen was checked into the NICU. The nurses and doctors that assisted us for the next week were amazing. They made sure we felt comfortable and reassured with the process. The first day in the NICU, Owen was hooked up to a CPAP machine which steadied out his breathing. After twenty-four hours, he was back to breathing normally on his own. The nurses took Owen's heel prick, and blood tests were run to determine if there were any other issues. The blood culture tests didn't find any bacteria, but his lungs were inflamed. It was decided that he would be put on antibiotics. Ben was able to stay the night at the hospital for the first two nights. It was really sweet because he had good bonding time with Owen before heading back to work for the week, and I got real sleep. My mom and I slept at the hospital the rest of the week. I started getting sick from mastitis and had a rough recovery. With the help of my family, Ben, and friends from church, dinner was brought to us for the week, and I was able to be with my sweet baby. Owen's round of antibiotics finished up in seven days, and we finally got to bring our perfectly sweet, healthy baby home. He truly is a bundle of joy.

Amber and Rachel's Home Birth

○ ○ ○ ○ ○ ○ ○ ○ ○ ○ ○ ○ ○ ○ ○ ○ ○ ○ ○

"While there were certainly some ups and downs being a same-sex couple during our pregnancy, I cherished the ups and refused to let the downs rule my life. Rachel and I lead a quiet and simple life. I wouldn't say we are activists, but we are advocates for peace and acceptance in that we live our lives without fear or hiding. Most importantly, we simply try to be kind and show the same acceptance and love to others that we desire to experience in this world."

—Amber, co-owner of Diversity Builder, Inc.

Nashville, Tennessee

My dreams were finally coming true. Rachel and I were married on October 15th, 2011, at Second Presbyterian Church in Nashville. It was an amazing day, only to be topped by our legal wedding on October 15th, 2012 in Boston, Massachusetts. We talked extensively about children, and while Rachel felt hesitant to become a parent late in life, she knew how important being a mother was to me and jumped into the conception process with total support and encouragement. We knew we wanted to try to keep the process as simple and natural as possible, so for six months we tried on our own at home.

I read every fertility book I could find: *Taking Charge of Your Fertility, Making Babies, The Tao of Fertility*, etc. I charted my BBT and did OPKs every month. I drank fertility tea and did regular fertility-friendly exercise and meditation. When I was still not pregnant after six months, we decided to go in for a fertility checkup just to make sure everything was okay. I passed every exam with flying colors. I was thirty-one years old, had more than perfect blood pressure and blood work, had regular periods, and a uterus that my doctor described as looking like the model on her desk.

She said she saw no reason why we shouldn't keep trying at home. Just to cover all our bases, we decided to run a newer test called AMH that would measure a different fertility hormone than the usual tests check for. I was devastated when I received the call that the test came back abnormal. My AMH level was well below what was considered the optimum level for conception, and there wasn't any way to correct it. The doctor said it was a good thing we were trying now, as I may not be able to have children at all in a short time.

We continued to push to conceive at home, and our doctor agreed to let us continue to try for another six months. We were prescribed Clomid to help stimulate my ovaries, and went back to the old fertility routine I had established. When another six months passed with no success, we went in for another visit with the doctor. While she tried to be encouraging, I was heartbroken and felt like a failure. For the first time in my life, I began to consider that maybe I wasn't meant to be a mother. That thought made me feel like I couldn't breathe. We decided at that appointment that we would switch fertility drugs to a newer drug called Femara and try for two more months at home. If that didn't work, then we would have to look at other, more invasive options. I left that meeting with little hope and lots of sadness.

The Femara made my cycle very different than usual, and we almost missed my ovulation day the next month. I started progesterone the day after ovulation and was instructed to stop taking it if I tested negative on my tenth day past ovulation (DPO). I had stopped taking pregnancy tests long ago, as every time I would see just one line it took a piece of me away. But on the tenth DPO, I pulled out a test from the back of the closet and took it. It was negative. I didn't even cry because I had nothing left. I stopped the progesterone and waited for the arrival of my period, expected on the fourteenth DPO. I had some major cramps and a little bloating on day thirteen, and knew I could expect my period at any time.

When the fourteenth day came and I still hadn't started my period, I grabbed another pregnancy test and headed to the bathroom. As I sat on the toilet and watched the second line come up, all I could do was stare at it. Rachel walked into the bathroom and saw me sitting there with the test in my hands and asked me what I was doing. All I could do was hand her the test. She looked at it, confused, and said that the second line was fainter than the first line. I tried to tell her that it didn't matter, that it was nothing like an ovulation predictor test, and a line was a line, but the words wouldn't come. When I was finally able to swallow the lump in my throat, I explained as best I could. After all the testing and emotion, she was skeptical and afraid to get her/our hopes up, so she immediately told me to take another test just to be sure. I sat and rocked back and forth on the toilet with my heart pounding, trying to squeeze out even a little urine for the second test since I had just gone to the bathroom. When that test also came back with a second line, the speechlessness was gone, and we both couldn't stop talking!

Shortly after, I began to panic, knowing that I was still supposed to be on the other medication if I tested positive, and I hadn't taken it in four days! So, I called my doctor through the on-call line (it was a Saturday) and fortunately, she called back quickly and told me to get right back on the medication and to not go off of it for twelve weeks. We scheduled an appointment for an ultrasound and blood work and got off the phone, but not before she gave us our first congratulations.

We had our blood work done the Wednesday and Friday following the test, and the numbers showed a progressively higher HCG, so pregnancy was confirmed.

We were finally pregnant!

We had an ultrasound at seven weeks and heard the heartbeat for the first time. We both cried. After having experienced my mother's miscarriage, we decided to only tell our closest friends until after the first trimester. The best part was telling my sister and my mom. We told my sister at six weeks by sending flowers to her at work with a card telling her what a wonderful aunt she was going to be to baby Stanton. We told my Mom a couple of days later on Easter Sunday. We made the official announcement to everyone else at twelve weeks, which just happened to be on Mother's Day.

Once we had confirmed our pregnancy, I drew on my past research and already had a plan in mind as to how I wanted to proceed with the prenatal care, birthing classes, and birth process. I knew that I wanted to have a vaginal, unmediated birth. I also knew I wanted to use a birthing method that would allow me to focus on what was happening with my body rather than one that used distraction, as well as something that would allow my wife to be as much a part of the birth process as possible. I felt that in order to accomplish those goals, I wanted to have a home birth with a midwife and use the Bradley method that teaches natural childbirth.

I shared my thoughts with Rachel and she was supportive right away. We both began researching midwives in the area and came up with a list. Being that we wanted Rachel to be very involved, we decided that she would make the initial calls to set up interview appointments. We sat down with our list and excitedly started at the top with our first call. My excitement quickly turned to doubt, embarrassment, and sadness when the first midwife turned us down for an interview with the explanation that her midwifery practice was a part of her spiritual ministry and therefore she was not comfortable working with a same-sex couple. While I had experienced similar situations when we were planning our wedding, this felt different because not only did it affect us as a couple, it was now affecting our child. As we went further down the list and were turned down again and again for the same reason, I felt utterly powerless and I began to wonder if we would be able to find a provider at all.

On the last call we made, the midwife again turned us down, but gave us a recommendation of someone that she felt might be a good fit. Her name was Jennifer. I was so disheartened at that point that I didn't even stay in the room when Rachel called her. When Rachel walked back in to the bedroom while on the phone, I tried to shoo her away, but she motioned to me that this call was different. I listened while Rachel made an appointment for an interview and immediately began researching Jennifer on the Internet.

When we met with Jennifer, we knew right away that she was going to be a good fit. She treated us like any other couple who might come through her practice, and never even mentioned the fact that our family was a little different than her usual clientele. She was knowledgeable, took the time to answer all of our questions, and seemed to like us, too. I again felt in charge of my pregnancy and birth.

We began our monthly visits and felt more comfortable with each appointment. During our third month, we moved from East Nashville to a house we had built in Hermitage. It felt like everything was coming together for our little family.

When it came time to sign up for our birth class, I was surprised when once again we were turned down for a class due to the fact that we were a same-sex couple. The instructor told us that a private class would be better for us, as she didn't feel that the other couples in a group class would accept us, and since it is such an intimate class, it would be very awkward for us and them. I felt the sense of powerlessness creeping back in, and I knew I had to keep trying or I would lose faith in the birth community all together. I knew of one other Bradley instructor in the area, Jeannie, so I wrote her and asked if she would allow a same-sex couple to be a part of her classes. She wrote back a kind message informing us that she expected parents to be supportive of other parents and that we would be welcome in her class. We started our class with a very diverse group of couples, and while there was some hesitation from a few of our classmates, we found that in general, we were all there for the same purpose, and that gave us a common bond.

While there were certainly some ups and downs being a same-sex couple during our pregnancy, I cherished the ups and refused to let the downs rule my life. Rachel and I lead a quiet and simple life. I wouldn't say we are activists, but we are advocates for peace and acceptance in that we live our lives without fear or hiding. Most importantly, we simply try to be kind and show the same acceptance and love to others that we desire to experience in this world.

At our thirty-six-week home visit, our midwife told us about a local artist who was creating a documentary with the intention of normalizing the home birth process. The artist asked Jennifer to collaborate with her and help her find couples to participate. The film would have interviews with couples planning a home birth before the birth, a video of the actual birth, and an after-the-birth interview. We were honored when Jennifer asked us to be involved. It was very exciting in that we would get to have our birth on film and be able to show some of the diversity of the home birth process. Rachel and I had actually tried to find some videos of same-sex couples who had home births and there were zero! Now, we had a chance to change that. In our before birth interview, we had a great time chatting with the artist and our midwife about home birth and our story. I look forward to being a part of the process and hopefully helping others out there know that there are other options for birth besides the hospital if they should want.

At thirty-eight weeks along, my pregnancy had been pretty unexceptional. While I felt queasiness from time to time in the first trimester, I never vomited. I was a bit tired, but nothing that felt unusual with packing and moving and all the transition happening in our lives at that time. My blood pressure has always been perfect and my blood and urine tests have tested normal. I didn't have any heartburn, constipation, or swelling. I didn't have any Braxton Hicks, and even my GBS test came back negative. Really, I didn't have any of the pregnancy symptoms that I've heard women complain about all my life. Other than my stomach becoming increasingly large and the fact that there was something moving around in there, I never physically felt any different.

Rachel and I decided not to find out the sex of our baby, so it was her job to "catch and call" as we like to say. We had gathered and organized all of our birth supplies by putting them in boxes in order of need and labeling the top of each box with what was inside. Our birth plans (home and transfer plans) were written and distributed. We tested the birth pool, attached the faucet adapter, and turned up the water heater. The nursery was mostly set up, all of the needed items for baby care put away, and car seats installed. I did still have several things on my to do list that I wanted to get done before the baby came, so I hoped the baby would stay in there for a couple more weeks.

I felt a little disconnected from the little one at times, and that made me feel guilty after everything we went through to get pregnant and how much I wanted to be a mother all of my life. I guess it was still hard for me to believe that there was really a baby in there and that at some point, it was going to come out!

I also really enjoyed my life the way it was at that moment. I liked spending time with my wife in our new home, traveling when we wanted, making our own schedules, and just spending time together. This was going to be a big change for the both of us. Don't get me wrong . . . I couldn't wait to meet this baby and I looked forward to all the smiles, love, and laughter I knew this little one would bring to our family. I knew we would be great parents, and that we complemented each other well when handling any sort of problem or conflict. I just didn't want to lose the connection we had to each other.

I became overwhelmed pretty easily those days. From cloth diapers to nursing bras, looking at all the options, learning the lingo, figuring out what I actually needed, and then finding the best deal all brought me to tears, and I am not one to cry often. Rachel was wonderful through it all, and I knew in my heart that as long as we were on the same team, there wasn't anything we couldn't handle.

November 19th, 2013: we were now 39+2 weeks along. Everything was about the same, meaning pretty unexceptional. I felt much more pressure in my nether regions when I walked around, bending over was nearly impossible, and my pelvis and hips were hurting a bit more, but nothing that was keeping me down. Rachel talked every day about how surprised she was by how active I still was. All of my friends and family thought I would be on bedrest by eight months due to my back surgery for a ruptured disc in 2010 and continued back issues (one reason I chose home birth). Thankfully, my back felt better than ever! I had very little pain (mostly a bit of sciatica in those last couple of months) and other than my back feeling tired here and there after a long day, I had no issues.

I also had allergy-related asthma that was very well controlled with daily allergy medication and an inhaler as needed. I go in once a year for a lung function test and to refill my inhaler, and this year my test came back better than ever at 103 percent! Everyone laughed because they thought for sure, being nine months pregnant, that I would show some kind of restriction with the pressure on my lungs. I said all along that I didn't feel any lung restriction except when exercising, and that test was confirmation.

I measured forty centimeters at my thirty-eight-week checkup and all the tests were normal. My blood pressure was a little higher than usual, but my blood pressure is usually low, so I was actually in the normal range. The midwife said the baby still hadn't dropped, but also said that it may not happen until I went into labor, and baby was still anterior, so that was great news.

I felt thankful that I had such an easy and enjoyable pregnancy. As Rachel is a bit older, this may be the only little one we have, so I am glad that I will be able to look back on this part of my life with a smile. I cried pretty easily those days, but they all seemed to be joyful tears over new homes, new babies, new marriages, etc. I loved seeing people happy and celebrating big events in their lives.

I also got emotional when I thought about handing our baby to Rachel for the first time. I had carried this little one for almost ten months now, and felt like I would be giving her a gift of some kind; something we both worked so hard for, but she hadn't yet been able to touch or really hold on to. I thought that moment would be one of the most exciting for me.

Still, the fact that I would be having this baby in the next couple of weeks was surreal to me. With no signs of labor or even labor preparation, it was easy for me to just think this baby would be in my belly for another few months! I knew in my head that labor was right around the corner, and for the first time, I stayed up with some anxiety and worry about the pain. The unknown was scary for me in general. Trying to prepare for an experience that is so unique for every woman is impossible, and I like to be prepared! But, I trusted my body and knew that it would all happen in the exact way and time that it should. I saw all the women in our birthing class having babies (some without any assistance!) and looked forward to that same feeling of accomplishment and pride in having completed the hard work of bringing a child into this world.

On Thanksgiving Day, November 28, 2013, and at forty weeks and five days pregnant, I still felt . . . fine. I did have a sense of being a bit more uncomfortable and having a harder time moving around, but otherwise everything was the same. I was also beginning to hate how huge I looked in every single photo that had been taken that day. Still, I hadn't had a single sign of labor, even though I'd been doing everything I knew to get things going for the last seven days: eating dates, taking evening primrose oil orally morning and night and vaginally at night, cinnamon morning and night, pineapple every day, walking and ball bouncing, sex, acupuncture every day, raspberry leaf tea, and foot massages and acupressure until my ankles were literally bruised. We even got permission from my midwife to try out the breast pump, as long as we did it exactly as she said. I had pumped lots of colostrum and still not had a single contraction.

I was feeling very down. My sister and niece were only in town for two more days, and if I don't have this baby before they left, they most likely wouldn't get to meet the baby for six months. That brings me to tears every time I think about it, even now while I am writing. My sister Andrea and I are very close. It is a bond that only identical twins can really understand. I wasn't able to be there for my niece's birth either, but I was on the phone and heard her first cry. Andrea was induced, so we had all scheduled our time to be there for the first several weeks after niece Aria's birth. My mom was there for the birth and first week after, my sisters-in-law were there for the second week, and I was there for the third week. We planned it that way, so that I could be the one to keep Aria for the first time overnight and give her the first bottle (my sister breastfed and didn't want to introduce the bottle until the third week). While I had been against any interventions for my own pregnancy and labor, this wait made me almost long for the easy scheduling of an induction. Then, maybe I wouldn't have felt so sad.

As a last-ditch effort to get contractions going, I took a two-mile walk down a very hilly road on midday Friday, November 29th, 2013. I walked mainly uphill for a mile and a half. No contractions came, but I was tired. Then my mom, sister, and I all went to acupuncture together. Still, nothing.

We had dinner at my dad's house (homemade sushi) and enjoyed some family time. I watched a movie with my niece and stayed up late talking with my sister.

Then, I finally gave in. Through tears I told my sister that she would have to meet my baby at another time as they were leaving at 6:00 a.m. on Sunday. We only had one more day together, and I didn't want to spend it trying to go into labor, only to have it start right as they were heading home. We both were sad, but planned to meet in Arkansas in January so she could see the baby. At 11:45 p.m. I wrote my midwife and told her we should go ahead and schedule a prenatal appointment for the next week. I ended my last sentence with a frown face. I crawled in bed around 12:30 a.m. and fell asleep quickly. It was a long, emotional day and I was ready for it to end.

At 2:30 a.m., I woke up. I was very groggy, and I couldn't figure out what had woken me from such a deep sleep. Then I felt the wetness pouring out from between my legs. I couldn't believe that I was peeing in the bed, but I had heard other women who were pregnant had peed on themselves from the pressure, so it seemed normal. I tried to stop the flow so I could go to the bathroom, and quickly realized that I couldn't. That was when I really woke up. I softly rubbed on my wife's shoulder and tried to wake her gently so she wouldn't be scared.

When she turned to me, I said, "Either I am peeing in the bed or my water just broke."

Her eyes opened wide and she whispered, "Well, you've never peed in the bed before, so it is probably your water breaking."

We both looked at each other for a minute without saying anything. I felt the excitement, fear, joy, and resolve all well up at once within both of us, and then I took action.

I told Rachel to smell the wet spot on the bed just to make sure it was what we thought it was, and she obliged with no questions. Once we confirmed that it wasn't urine on the sheets, I told her to go upstairs and wake up my sister. (She later told me that when she woke Andrea up and told her my water broke that my sister's first words were, "Are you kidding?")

While I was waiting, I began to think about what needed to happen next. When Andrea and Rachel came back downstairs, I asked them to get a pad and help me get to the bathroom, as fluid was still coming out of me, and I didn't want to get it on the carpet. I put the pad between my legs, waddled to the bathroom, and sat on the toilet. I told Rachel to call Jennifer, and she did. Jennifer asked if the fluid was clear and we confirmed that it was. She then asked if I was having any contractions. I wasn't.

Jennifer's next words made me laugh, "Well, then I suggest you go back to sleep and try to get some rest until the contractions start."

My sister called my mom and dad and texted our best friends to let them know that my water had broken. Then, as Rachel had learned in our Bradley class, she calmly took control and insisted that we all try to get some rest while we could. She knew two hours of sleep would not be enough to get me through what was about to happen. My sister went out to sleep on the couch in the living room, and we laid down some pads on the wet sheets and snuggled in under the covers. It took me a while to relax, but I finally fell asleep listening to the even sounds of Rachel's breath.

It seemed like I had just drifted off when I woke up to what felt like period cramps. It only lasted a brief moment, so I ignored it and tried to go back to sleep, but it happened again a very short time after. When the third round happened shortly after, I grabbed my phone. It was 3:30 in the morning. I hadn't even been able to sleep for more than fifteen minutes. I started timing the cramps with my phone app and realized that they had been as close together as I thought. They were only five minutes apart. I kept timing them over the next thirty minutes and knew that I wasn't going to be able to go back to sleep.

At 4:00 a.m., I woke Rachel again and told her that contractions had started and while not really painful yet, were already pretty close and regular. My sister, who was having a hard time going back to sleep herself, heard us talking and came in the room. Knowing that sleep wasn't going to happen for me, I decided to go ahead and get up and start on my list of things I wanted to do before Jennifer came. Determined not to poop in the birthing pool, I asked them to help me do an enema, as I had never done

one before. We all laughed throughout the entire process and the laughter helped to relieve some of the anxiety I was beginning to feel. My sister then told Rachel that she would stay up with me and for her to try to go back to sleep. I got in the shower and shaved my legs while my sister sat outside, timing my contractions. They were never longer than five minutes apart, but were very inconsistent in length and strength.

At 6:00 a.m., we decided to wake Rachel again as the contractions were around three minutes apart, albeit inconsistent. We called our midwife and left a message when she didn't answer. Rachel continued to try to get in touch with her over the next couple of hours. Andrea and Rachel both started working on their to-do lists that I had made for them: setting up my birth stations, cleaning out the bathtub, putting out the home birth supply boxes, setting up the birth pool, emptying all the trash cans throughout the house, etc. We called my mom to let her know that I was in labor and she immediately set about getting ready to come.

Around 8:00 a.m. my contractions were getting stronger, so I got in the tub to get warm and ease some of the pain. I called my close friends to let them know and had to put the phone down to get through a contraction. At about 8:30 a.m. my midwife called and was frantic. Apparently, the cell towers were down in her part of town and she hadn't received any of the calls or texts we had sent since the first one. When the towers went up, all the voicemails and texts came through and she thought she had missed the birth. We assured her that she hadn't, but encouraged her to come on over.

Jennifer arrived about an hour later. By that time, I was out of the tub and sitting on the yoga ball trying to relax through the cramping. We were chatting and I had to stop talking to get through a contraction. Based on that and the timing of the contractions, Jennifer asked to check me as she thought I might be going into transition. When she completed her check, and told me that I was only at three centimeters, I said the one and only curse word I would say throughout my labor, a loud and resounding, "*Sh*t*."

Shortly thereafter, I vomited and moved into a state of what I can only describe as delirium. I went so deep inside myself that I couldn't even hear what was going on around me. I was exhausted, and the pain during each contraction was so much more than I could have ever imagined. It hurt to even breathe. I laid on the bed and fell asleep between each contraction, but they were so close together that it didn't allow me much time to rest.

As the day progressed, Jennifer told Rachel that I could stay on the bed and rest if I wanted, but it would most likely take longer than if I got up and moved around. Rachel came to me and asked, "Do you want to rest or do you want to get it over with?" I wanted to get it over with! I tried to walk around, but the pain of one contraction would barely go away before another started. Our baby's godmothers arrived around noon. They had sped from Asheville to Nashville hoping to make it in time for the birth. They set up the massage table and moved me to the living room so that Robin (a certified masseuse) could try to massage me through the contractions.

At some point, Jennifer checked me again and said that I was at seven centimeters and could get in the birth pool if I wanted. I was so ready for some relief that I was willing to try anything. I got in the pool, but couldn't find a comfortable position. I was either too low in the water and felt like I was going to drown or too high and felt too cold. I got on my hands and knees for a while, but when I tried to put my head on the side of the tub, the side would bend down and I would worry about the water getting on the carpet. Eventually, Robin and Abbey came over to the side and held me up under my arms while squatting next to the tub. Sometimes they would hold me together, sometimes they would switch off, but for over an hour at least one of them held me in their arms. Looking back, I don't know how they did it.

It was during that time that Jennifer became concerned about my breathing and kept telling me to breathe slower and deeper, but I physically felt like I couldn't. Breathing hurt and any time I would breathe in deep, the pain would just skyrocket. My sister came to my side and started breathing deeply in my ear and I automatically started to match her breaths without even knowing it. It was during that time that I realized if I would bear down just a bit when a contraction would hit that it would help ease the pain. Jennifer noticed and checked me again. She said that I had a bit of a cervical lip and for me not to do any pushing yet because she was trying to prevent pressure on that lip. Every time she or anyone else spoke to me, they had to say it twice, because the first time they said it I wouldn't hear it. I was in a trancelike state that was anything but peaceful. It was very hard not to bear down when I knew that it would help the pain so much, but I did my best to listen and control myself.

During my time in the pool someone asked me how I was doing and I remember answering that I was ready to be done. Everyone kind of giggled and while I knew it was probably lighthearted, the sound made me want to cry. I was so tired and in so much pain that I couldn't imagine ever being able to laugh again. If I had been anywhere near able, I would have probably ordered everyone out of the room at that point so that I could have a little breakdown, but I couldn't even speak.

After a few more contractions, I turned again on my hands and knees trying to do anything to help the pain. Jennifer told Rachel that if I stayed in that position that it would be okay for me to push when I felt like I needed to push. Rachel came to my head and whispered what Jennifer had said to her. I was relieved and decided to bear down gently like I had been doing before when the next contraction came.

But when the next contraction came and I started to push gently, it felt like something took over my body and started pushing as hard as possible. I felt warm water being forced out of my vagina at such a high speed that it almost burned. I panicked and started yelling that I couldn't help it, that it just happened. Jennifer calmed me down and told me that it was just my body telling me it was time to start pushing. Knowing that the end was coming was such a relief. Instead of just having to sit and wait through each contraction, I could *do* something.

That focus was all I needed. With each contraction, I pushed and felt the baby's head come down the canal. When the contraction was over, I would feel the head move back up and I told myself that was how it was supposed to be. I was very nervous about tearing, and I knew that if I would allow the baby to come down further each time and not rush, that it would help give my body time to stretch and accommodate the baby's head. Jennifer encouraged me by telling me that I was a great pusher and that I had plenty of room for the baby to come out. After a few contractions, Jennifer suggested I squat to try to get the baby's head out. Sure enough, with the next contraction his head popped right out. I let out a cry because I was so surprised that it came out. I had no idea it was so close!

I went back to my hands and knees and Jennifer tried to pull the baby out, but it hurt so badly that I cried out and she stopped. As soon as the next contraction came, he was out and Jennifer placed the baby in Rachel's hands. Being on my hands and knees I couldn't see the baby, but I knew it had been born. Jennifer helped me turn around without disturbing the cord and then placed the baby on my chest. When the baby started crying it was a beautiful sound, but all I could think was that I felt like crying too. I was totally spent.

Soon after someone mentioned something about the baby being a girl and everyone erupted with excitement. Shortly after, Jennifer tried to confirm the sex with Rachel, but quickly realized that there had been a big miscommunication and no one really knew what sex the baby was! I took off the towels and did a quick check myself finding that the baby was *all* boy. Everyone laughed, and that time I didn't mind. Our son was here. Ryman Neile Stanton. Born at 3:55 p.m. at seven pounds, one ounce, nineteen inches long after only fifteen minutes of pushing.

It took almost an hour (and fifteen minutes of squatting beside the bed, determined not to have Pitocin) for me to deliver the placenta and even longer to have any sort of bleeding. I had no tearing and no pain. After a bit, I took a shower and we all ate the roast that had been cooking since that morning (one of the jobs on my mom's labor to do list). One by one my family members (dad, stepdad, niece, brother-in-law, etc.) came to get a look at our newest family member. Jennifer and her assistant changed the sheets and cleaned up our bedroom so that we could all get some good rest that evening. Then we all gathered in the living room laughing, talking, and enjoying each other's company until one by one everyone left or went to their room and our little family was together for the first time as a threesome.

The birth experience was one of the hardest things I have ever done in my life. I came away telling Rachel that I didn't know if I could ever give birth again. The pain and exhaustion were overwhelming. But honestly, I can't imagine birthing any other way. Being in my own safe space with my family and friends helping to take care of me, and each other, was a powerful and soul changing event that I hope to one day be able to have again.

A Single Mom Surrounded
by Supportive Women

○ ○ ○ ○ ○ ○ ○ ○ ○ ● ● ● ● ● ○ (○

"I want mamas to know that home birth isn't only for happily married couples. It's important to share that having a baby with a supportive group of family and/or friends or all by yourself can be just as beautiful and impacting. There really is no cookie-cutter or picture perfect birth story. Each of my three children has a different birth story and each one has impacted me differently, changing me as a mama and human being."

—Terra, registered nurse
Vancouver, Washington

I have been pregnant five times and delivered three babies. Heather, my first, was born in the hospital—not a great experience. The estimated due date for Heather was July 27th, and by the time I was approaching two weeks "overdue" my doctor told me if I happened to be out of network when I went into labor, my insurance wouldn't cover her birth. She also told me that it's dangerous for my baby to be in the womb for too long, so induction was the best, safest option. I wanted the best and safest situation for my baby, plus, I was young and unaware of factors that can affect the length of pregnancy (e.g., the length of my menstrual cycle, or my health at the time of conception). So, naturally, I agreed to be induced. It's important to note that even with my original plan of having a hospital birth, I wanted to avoid an epidural or any other interventions that might negatively affect my baby. I signed my husband at the time and myself up for a Bradley Method birth class. However, it was a thirty-minute drive from our house, and he had to get up early for work, so he didn't want to go after the first class. Instead of being well-prepared for a natural birth, I felt ill prepared for *any* birth!

On August 10th, I checked in for my induction at seven in the morning. I was told that we'd start easy with misoprostol to soften my cervix with the goal/hope that my body would be inspired to go into labor. That didn't work. The next step was Pitocin, which I really didn't want, but I was told that if my own laboring efforts didn't kick in I could decide if I wanted to go home. By the end of that day, I had barely dilated and my body was not participating in the process at all. But when the question of home or baby tonight came up, I was too exhausted to say no. Looking back, whether or not they meant to, it feels like I was scammed! Once I signed on to the "we're having a baby tonight!" plan, the Pitocin route became a lot more aggressive.

I felt sick. I was having massive contractions, and still not progressing. With that medication, I was begging for anything that could help with the pain I was feeling. I was told I wasn't dilated enough for an epidural, so they gave me a medication that basically knocked me out between contractions, but let me feel the full force of each Pitocin-laced contraction. I was finally "barely a three" (three centimeters dilated) later that evening and was told I could have an epidural if I wanted one. Of course, I jumped on that offer—even though it would become something I'd feel guilty about later on—and was soon resting. It wasn't long after that that I embarrassingly told the nurse, "I think I need to poop!" She told me that was a good sign and gloved up to check my progress. As soon as she went to check she said, "Oh my gosh! There's the head!" The doctor came in and began directing my pushing, which I couldn't feel at all due to the epidural. It was a very out of control feeling, because no matter what they were telling me, I didn't know how to physically duplicate what was being required.

During this time, I let the doctor know I really didn't want an episiotomy. I had learned from my mom's visual example of trying to tear an intact T-shirt vs. Trying to tear a T-shirt with a little snip in it that letting my skin stretch and maybe have a tiny tear was better than an episiotomy and possible tear on top of that. What I didn't realize is that going from three centimeters to delivery in thirty to forty minutes was far less time than I needed to keep my perineum intact and I ended up tearing badly. What made it worse was that the doctor felt it was necessary to sarcastically let me know, "You got the tear you wanted." Holding my baby was indescribable, but the impending pain and complications from delivery and nursing difficulties were *not* a fair trade!

A little over a week later I got up too quickly and reopened my tear.

Already an incredibly painful experience, when I was examined at the urgent care clinic the doctor blurted out, "Oh my God, the vagina is such a dirty hole! You're totally infected." Embarrassed and completely horrified at the medications she prescribed, I broke down crying several times that day alone.

As it turns out, during the recommended follow-up appointment the next day my normal ob-gyn matter-of-factly said, "You're not infected at all. Your stitches tore out." This whole experience was major fuel on my home birthing mama fire! I wanted a different experience with my next pregnancies, so I had John and Jack at home with the midwife who delivered me in 1979! She was also the midwife for two of my siblings and present for the Cesarean birth of my youngest brother. Already having one baby at home, I knew I definitely wanted to have Jack at home, too. I believed it was best for us, and a peaceful environment was exceptionally important to me, as well. My husband at the time, Nate, and I had separated around twelve weeks into my pregnancy, and while I thought things were going to get better and that surely by the time I was in maternity clothes or autumn rolled around we'd be back together, we weren't. Our relationship had become slowly more strained and stressful. I needed peace and support. That's what this home birth provided.

The most challenging part of my decision to have Jack at home was related to my separation from Nate and the general uncertainty in my life. Heather (seven years old), John (three years old), and I were living in my parents' house at the time. Living with other people is always complicated, and my situation was no exception. I heard messages from some that Nate should absolutely not be present at Jack's birth, and the opposite, that because he's the father he has a right to be there. I wanted this to be easy, but it became apparent that there wasn't a right or wrong answer and that the most powerful thing I could do was to independently decide what was best for my family and then act.

Thankfully, they were completely supportive of me having a home birth in their home. However, once the final baby countdown began, I really had to evaluate whether it was best for me to have Nate present at Jack's birth or not. Life was very stressful at the time, and I wanted to bring my baby into a peaceful environment. In addition, between John's birth and Jack's pregnancy I had had two miscarriages, and I wasn't one hundred percent sure they weren't due to something I had or hadn't done. Not that I did anything different then before; I was really examining what the best, safest plan of action would be for this pregnancy.

I sailed through the pregnancy without complications, simply waiting for labor to begin. Contractions started around 1:00 p.m., so I tried the "eat it off, walk it off, sleep it off" technique to see if I could make labor stop. When I realized that contractions were coming consistently every six minutes, I knew this was the real deal. By 3:00 p.m. my contractions were coming every four to five minutes and lasting one minute. I had also started leaking a clear to pinkish fluid, so I called my midwife. My parents began inflating and filling the birthing tub while my sister went to pick my seven-year-old daughter up from school. I was in the tub as soon as it was filled, and our midwife, Mary, arrived at 3:45 that afternoon. At 4:00 p.m., Mary checked my cervix and told me I was only about three and a half centimeters dilated, which was very disappointing, as I was at three centimeters several days before (labor false alarm!).

I kept laboring in the tub, just trying to stay relaxed so my body could work. I drank some smoothie, got up and went to the bathroom, but came right back to the tub. The contractions were so intense; I just knew they had to be doing something, so I asked Mary to check me again. It had been one and a half hours since she last checked my cervix, and I anticipated she'd tell me I was an eight or maybe a nine; however, as she was checking I had a feeling I was wrong.

Mary said, "Well . . ."

I interrupted, saying, "Just tell my I'm not still a three."

Mary laughed and said, "Well, you're not a three, but you are a four!"

At that, I was done with the pool. I decided to walk around to see if that would help. I thought it'd be nice to go visit with people upstairs, but that didn't help either. I went back downstairs where I ran into Pita. I imagine she could see that I needed help directing my body. She suggested I bend at the waist, supporting myself on the arms of a rocking chair where I could rock standing up and let my belly hang free during the contractions. Her directions were incredibly calming; it was as if I obeyed her commands without having to think of how to do it. This was exceptionally helpful, as I believe I was in transition at that point.

I really wanted to get off my feet and had heard that sitting backwards on a toilet with a pillow on the tank for support was a very comfortable way to labor. I quickly realized the word "comfortable" was not an accurate description of the position, but it felt nice to be off my feet. It crossed my mind to try and secretly do some mini pushes while I was on the toilet in hopes that it would relieve a little of the pain I was feeling. On my second "mini push" at 6:18 p.m., my water broke. The sensation in my pelvis changed and I knew it was baby-time!

I walked out of the bathroom bow-legged like an old cowgirl, and told Kelly (my future sister-in-law), "Baby's comin'!"

She ran upstairs and delivered the news to the rest of those waiting while I waddled back to the tub. I got in a hands and knees position, as this worked so well with my last baby, and I listened to Pita coach me through pushing. Jack was born five minutes later at 6:23 in the evening.

I held Jack in the tub surrounded by those I love and cherish. My midwife swaddled my baby and handed him to my mom while I quickly showered. Now in my room, I was surrounded again by loved ones who were raising glasses of champagne, imprinting their hearts' desires for Jack and celebrating his arrival. I drank in the beauty of my perfectly formed nine-pound baby boy and the love surrounding us. It wasn't the audience I thought I would have for Jack's birth, but it was the environment I needed at that moment.

A Doula on Skype!

○ ○ ○ ○ ○ ○ ○ ○ ○ ○ ○ ○ ○ ○ ○ ○ ○ ○

"I have been with Selena and Jason since the beginning of their journey to conceive. I am married to Selena's brother, and although we are not related by blood, we consider each other sisters. Selena and I share a special bond for many reasons, and supporting each other through trying to conceive only deepened that shared bond."

—Caitlin, certified birth doula
San Antonio, Texas

After years of trying to conceive, Selena and Jason were getting ready to give up. I convinced Selena that she should contact a doctor and see if there were any issues stopping her from being able to get pregnant. They did all the testing, but didn't receive any answers except that her preexisting medical conditions (polycystic ovary syndrome, pancreatitis, and interstitial cystitis) gave her only a 2 percent chance of getting pregnant.

Month after month we worked through the disappointment, anger, sadness, and confusion of yet another negative pregnancy test. Struggling with infertility comes with battles all its own. Not only do you have to deal with being let down every month, you also have to deal with people asking questions like, "When are you having a baby?" When you tell them you've been working on it and it's just not happening, those same people are really quick to move on to saying how you should enjoy the life you have and that everything happens for a reason. Although well meaning, these comments can often lead to more frustration.

Selena decided that they were going to take a break from trying to conceive for a few months as the emotions were really starting to take a toll on her day-to-day life. Now, if you've ever known anyone struggling to get pregnant, you know that they never really take a break. They always think about timing intercourse, what time of the month it is, when their period is going to come, and when it's a day late. Inevitably, they start thinking about when they can take a pregnancy test.

I was still living in Germany at this point and Selena was in California, so my nights were her afternoons. One night, later than I would normally be awake, I checked my phone and saw a missed call and fifteen text messages asking me to call as soon as I could. I got up and FaceTimed her with one eye half open. The grin was huge; a smile from ear to ear. I was told to hang on while she went in the other room, since she was still at work. Next thing I knew, there was a little white stick blurringly being shoved in the camera while she fumbled to get the test results in the right spot so I could see them. And then she said it. The words we had been waiting years to hear finally came out of her mouth.

"I'm pregnant!"

The tears started to flow.

Knowing the feelings that come with finally getting pregnant after years of being unsuccessful, there was still a lot to work through. There were so many thoughts of *what am I going to do? What if it doesn't work out? What if I can't do this? What if I'm a bad mom?* The feelings just kept coming, and coming, and coming. We worked through them all, every single day.

The pregnancy was fairly smooth sailing with a few minor bumps in the road. Not knowing what pains were normal really worried Selena. I tried to be as reassuring as I could, but being all the way in Germany, and not knowing enough about her preexisting conditions, there wasn't a lot I could say for sure. Just before the twenty-week mark, she started experiencing abdominal pain that lasted for a long time, leaving her nauseous, unable to walk, feeling terrified, and asking me what to do. I'm very big on trusting your intuition. We talked about how if she was worried enough to be asking me what she should do, then she should be going to the emergency room (ER). It's typical hospital policy that pregnant women go to the ER instead of Labor and Delivery before the twenty-week mark as the pregnancy isn't considered viable until you are twenty weeks. Of course, upon getting to the ER she was put on a list with everyone else there waiting to see a doctor. After waiting and waiting, she was finally seen. They decided that she was having some minor contractions but because she wasn't yet twenty weeks, there was nothing they could do for her. If she had been just a few more days into her pregnancy, she would have been admitted to labor and delivery and given medication to stop the contractions. They sent her home with orders to rest and simply "wait and see."

Everything worked out, and that incident was really the only major issue during her pregnancy, with an exception of the disagreements with her hospital obstetrician (OB). Selena had wanted a birth on the more natural side. Hospitals, needles, medications, etc., just didn't really appeal to her. They checked out the local birth center but decided that the out-of-pocket fee was too much. Their next discussion was a home birth with a midwife. Jason was not keen on this idea as his children from a previous relationship were born in the hospital, and his daughter was born several weeks early and needed to stay in the NICU. Although he didn't agree with a home birth, he agreed to meet with the midwife. The meeting didn't go very well. He didn't go into the meeting with an open mind and still saw the hospital as the place to be when having a baby.

Selena, disappointed, continued her prenatal care at the hospital. We went over making sure she told the OB of her birth goals, explaining to them about her fear of needles and the zillion other things we had discussed. At this appointment, she realized that she was just going to be pushed through the Labor and Delivery ward as if she were just another animal in a herd of cattle. This feeling only made her disappointment grow. Her confidence in the ability to birth her baby the way she wanted was gone. She was suddenly terrified of giving birth.

After another mishap with the hospital staff, Selena decided she'd had enough. She canceled all of her remaining prenatal appointments and kept telling me that she would just do this at home by herself. She knew that Jason would never go for the home birth so she would just have to "accidentally" have the baby at home. I urged her to talk to Jason and explain what happened at her last doctor's appointment and revisit the option to have a midwife at home. She complained to me and said there was no way he would go for it, but we talked about how she would only know if she tried. Selena ended up talking to Jason about her appointment, and he agreed to meet with the midwife again; this time keeping an open mind. Selena also had Jason watch *The Business of Being Born*. The film resonated with him, and his mind became more open to the idea of home birth.

This second meeting with the midwife went great. Jason was able to ask all the questions he had and agreed that this seemed like a better option for their family. I remember waking up to a text that read "Guess who's having a home birth?" That was a level of excitement I hadn't seen for quite a while. At thirty-two weeks pregnant, Selena switched to midwifery care, and it seemed to change her whole outlook on labor and delivery.

Time seemed to pass significantly faster after Selena's decision to have a home birth. Selena was excited to have prenatal meetings with her midwife, which made the week go by quicker. Next thing she knew, the birth pool was being delivered and it was time to order the birth kit as she was finally cleared for her home birth (in California, you are not "cleared" to have a home birth until you reach at least thirty-seven weeks' gestation, as that is when the likelihood of the NICU being a necessity goes down). When Selena was thirty-nine weeks, she decided that she was ready to go on maternity leave. Time slowed down again. Sitting and waiting is hard. Thirty-nine weeks quickly turned into forty. Forty weeks turned into forty-one.

At about forty weeks and two days, Selena was talking to her midwife about natural induction methods. She was instructed to start taking black and blue cohosh to help bring on contractions. It was also suggested that she start drinking red raspberry leaf tea and begin using a breast pump to stimulate contractions. None of this did anything. There were no contractions, no signs of early labor, nothing to give Selena any hope that labor was coming any time soon.

When forty-one weeks rolled around, Selena started to panic, thinking that she wasn't going to get her home birth since most midwives can't deliver you past forty-two weeks. She spent her days worrying that all this fighting to get her dream birth would be for nothing. I had a strong feeling that her due date was wrong. I remember her telling me that her due date was one thing and then after another ultrasound it was changed. The hospital was going off of the earlier date. At her next prenatal appointment with her midwife, she brought up the possibility of her due date being wrong. They reviewed her paperwork and decided that she was not forty-one weeks pregnant, but was really only forty weeks pregnant. This would give Selena another two weeks to deliver, which made everyone feel a little bit better.

Memorial Day was approaching, and that was the day Jason was supposed to help their midwife move. We kept making jokes that because they had made plans for that day, that was the day baby would decide to come. On May 29th, Selena finally took my advice to go swimming. Swimming is really beneficial when you're pregnant since it is so low impact and the water helps lift some of the pressure from the weight of the baby. Since you're out moving and the water lifts your belly, it helps to give baby the opportunity to get into a better position. That night before bed, Selena also put castor oil and clary sage oil on her belly. This was a suggestion from the midwife which would help bring on contractions if her body was finally ready.

Around 6:30 in the morning my time (4:30 a.m. in California), I got a message from Selena that read, "I'm in labor." At this time, Selena will take over writing the birth story.

I can remember waking up around 2 a.m. PST with the need to void my bladder, again. I got up, went to the bathroom, and began feeling some pretty intense cramps. Not thinking too much about it, I crawled back to bed. Approximately thirty minutes later, I had to void again and the cramping was getting worse. After I wiped I saw it: bloody show! The cramping was pretty intense by this point. I went back to my bedroom and bent over the side of the bed. I began to rock my hips and breathe slow and deep. This lasted another half hour before I knew it was really time. Finally!

I reached over the bed, grabbed Jason's leg, and said, "Babe, this is it, it's happening." Jason opened his eyes and said, "Contractions?"

"Yup," was all I could get out.

"How far apart?"

"No idea, but it hurts."

Jason sat up with me until I started moaning.

Around 4:15 a.m. Jason said, "Call the midwife, and let her know what's happening."

It was so early in the morning that I didn't want to wake her, so I sent her a text even though I knew she would be ticked at me for not sending her a page. When a few minutes went by I texted my other midwife, Laura, as well. She called me. I told her what was happening.

Laura replied, "Call Claudette, let her know we are having a baby today, mama! I will see you soon."

Ugh. I didn't want to wake Claudette! Even so, I called her and woke her up.

"Mmm, hello?"

"Claudette, it's Selena. I'm having contractions and a bloody show."

"How far apart are the contractions?"

"I don't know, every few minutes, but it's really hurting bad." Me breathing.

"Okay, I can hear that the contraction is only lasting about twenty to thirty seconds. Lay down, get the heating pad out, and call me when the contraction lasts sixty seconds."

*Well, sh*t,* I remember thinking. I was in so much pain that I thought the baby was coming right now. "Alright, I think I am going to take a warm shower, too, Claudette."

"That's good, do that. Call me back. I'll see you soon. This is your first baby, we have lots of time."

In my head: *no! There's no way there's time. He's coming now. This pain is so intense!* After I got off the phone, I told Jason what was happening. He helped get me set up in bed with the heating pad. Then he went downstairs to straighten up and prepare for the birth. At this point I messaged Caitlin, our doula, on Facebook. (I didn't want to wake her up yet either.) After that, I jumped in the shower and rested my head against the wall as the contractions began to grow stronger. With each contraction, I would vomit. I couldn't control it. Then I would get sleepy and nod off. Knowing this was dangerous, since I was standing up in the shower, I decided to get out and lay back in bed with the heating pad. However, before I could get to my bed, I landed my behind straight on the toilet. Oh no. Diarrhea. Diarrhea and vomiting. How could it be that I am in this much pain and having issues already? I thought I would be able to sleep, relax, maybe eat. Nope. This birth was going to be hardcore from the start.

Jason came upstairs to check on me once I was able to stumble back into the bed. He asked how I was doing, and I told him I wanted him to bring me my mascara, that I at least needed to put some of my face on.

He said, "No you don't, that is ridiculous. You don't need to put make-up on, just relax." Boy, was I mad. I knew I looked like crap and man, did I feel like crap! However, at this point, the pain was so insane that I didn't have the energy to argue. The sun had begun to come out. That irritated me, too. I was so hoping to have a night birth, in the dark. It was nearly summer in Santa Rosa, and it was too damn hot in our apartment with no air conditioning. Lying in bed, I looked down at my phone and realized I was having contractions lasting longer than 60 seconds. I called Claudette, and she said she would be on her way shortly and for me to keep breathing and resting. Easy for her to say (sorry, Claudette!).

At approximately 7:30 a.m., my strong and powerful midwife, Claudette, came in. Relief! She came upstairs, looked me in the face, and said, "Oh yeah, hunny, you're gonna feel all of it. You can do anything for sixty seconds, remember that. Do you want me to check you to see how far we are?"

Pretty sure I mumbled, "Yes please."

"Yup, you're at about a four and totally effaced."

Only a four? No, I needed this over now, but my son and my body had other plans for me that day. Claudette said we still had some ways to go and decided she was going to go and get the moving truck (even though Jason couldn't help because I was fixin' to have a baby). She said she would be back soon and that Laura was on the way, too. I laid there in disbelief. My body continued to "freak out" as I call it: vomit, diarrhea, moan. I kept telling myself to breathe and go with the contraction and rock. Psh. Not that easy once you're in the moment.

Laura came in around 8:30 in the morning. She came up the stairs to find me laying on the floor, on my side, and gripping the legs of my soon to be born son's swing.

Laura sat next to me and rubbed my legs (thankfully, I had shaved the day before) and said softly, "How's it going, mama?"

I let out a long and low moan. She told me I was doing a great job. My body was able to let me mutter the words "pain and pool." Laura asked me if I wanted to get in the birth tub. Oh, heck yes, I did.

I could hear Jason say from downstairs, "I'm filling it now."

He was doing so great. I couldn't have asked for a better birth partner.

Laura helped me hobble down the stairs and into the tub. Relief! Holy moly, that warm, wonderful water took my pain from about an eight to a five. Whew! I looked over and saw my sister-in-law and "virtual doula" looking at me through the screen of Jason's computer. I knew she had texted me when I was upstairs, but I was in so much pain that I couldn't even properly respond. Jason knew how important she was to my birth plan, so he called her up and got her on FaceTime. Jason also was able to call Nana, my grandmother, to tell her we were going to be having a baby that day. I had told Jason that Nana was the first call to make no matter what happened and he kept his promise to notify her first.

The next hours are still a blur. I can't remember everything. My best friend, Alicia, showed up to help the midwives and Jason. While laboring in the tub I would pass out between contractions. Jason would nudge the side of the tub and tell me I was snoring while Alicia would tell him to leave me alone, because I needed rest. It felt strange sitting in the tub, waiting for my body to decide the right time for our baby, Blaine, to come out. It was also strange knowing that these people were staring at me, waiting and wondering, as well.

Around noon, I think, Claudette wanted me to go upstairs and try to labor in bed, because she was afraid labor was stalling from the tub.

I had continued to throw up while in the birth tub, and I was becoming dehydrated, so we hobbled up the stairs to the bed. Laura came with the fan, because my apartment was getting to be like the third level of Hell, it was so hot. Once we all got upstairs, Claudette checked my cervix. I was dilated to an eight in the front and a ten in the back. She said this happens to moms who have scar tissue and that I needed to NOT push when I had a contraction. This was tricky as I was feeling the need to push. With the next contraction, Claudette had to manually open my cervix. My back labor was so intense, and I was still vomiting, (Alicia was trying to feed me popsicles with little success) so I was given lime-flavored coconut water (so gross). My husband was putting the straw in my mouth and telling me to drink. Yuck.

Here's the picture of my bedroom at this time: Claudette's hand in my vagina, opening my cervix, Alicia holding my hand, Laura positioning the fan and wiping me because I was still having bowel movements, as well, Jason trying to feed me the coconut water, and me looking around for the computer.

"Jason, where is Caitlin?" I asked.

"Downstairs, babe."

"Go get her. I need her."

The next time I looked over, there was the MacBook with Caitlin smiling at me. I had all the most important people to me at that time, in my bed with me. Claudette kept telling me not to push, but it was hard not to. My body was automatically pushing. She told me that my cervix could swell up and we would have to start all over again. Very frustrating. Eventually, it grew too hot upstairs, and I was needing the bathroom again. Everyone decided a break would be good, and Claudette wanted me to come downstairs after bathroom time and try pushing on the laboring stool.

Here we go again. When I was done in the bathroom, I went to go back downstairs. One step and *boom*! Major contraction.

Alicia said, "Oh no, Selena, don't have this baby on the stairs, please don't have the baby on the stairs!"

Claudette, from the bottom of the stairs said, "No this is great! Push him out. Push, Selena, it's okay."

Well, I pushed, and he stayed in, so I went down the stairs again and onto the birth stool. Jason was over by the computer, talking to Caitlin. I didn't know it at the time, but apparently, he was getting worried that the midwives weren't telling him something was wrong. Caitlin was doing her doula thing and calming him, which I greatly appreciated. Onto the birth stool . . . nope. Hated that thing. The back labor was too intense, and I needed to lay down. Claudette wanted me to hang onto a sheet over my stair rails and pull. No effing way. Me standing up was *not* going to happen. It was too painful, and I was exhausted and hot. So, I laid on the carpet. Claudette shot some B12 into my thigh to keep me going, Jason was feeding me the stupid coconut water, which at this point, was too hot, and I was so pissed he was making me drink it.

After 3:00 p.m., I was on my back on my living room floor. Jason was holding one leg and Alicia the other. Midwife Claudette had me playing tug of war with a sheet, and Midwife Laura was snapping photos and wiping my rear end. Joy! I can't remember the point of the tug of war, but I remember Alicia telling me she could see Blaine's hair. I'm pretty sure I tried to say *pull him out, then*, but maybe that was just in my mind. Talking was so hard during labor, I really couldn't believe how hard it was. The midwives had me try the birth stool again. No way. That was so uncomfortable and hurt my rear end. After this and more tug of war, Alicia told me she had to get home to her babies. After Alicia told me she loved me and then left, I laid on my side on the floor, and it felt like I was convulsing. Claudette allowed me to lay there for a moment while she talked to Laura. I'm sure they were concerned about what was going on with my body and what the next step was to get Blaine out. I could feel my body changing, though. I can't explain it.

I shouted, "I need to f*cking push!"

And Claudette said, "Do it!"

I laid on my side and pushed hard. I could feel something move.

I sat up and said, "I need to get back in the pool, I can't do this without the pool."

I got into the pool, bent over the side on my hands and knees, and pushed with each contraction. These pushes felt different. The midwives were also in the kitchen, leaving me to do my thing, which helped. Jason stayed by my side, concerned. At one point, I pushed and told Claudette that something felt different. I rolled onto my butt, spread my legs, and pushed again. I was exhausted. It felt like I couldn't go on, and I needed a break.

Claudette looked at Laura and then at me and said, "Okay. You've been pushing for four hours. If the baby isn't born in the next thirty minutes, we need to go to the hospital; it isn't safe for him."

No! I wanted my son born at home in this stupid tub, no freaking way was I going to a hospital. Then I thought to myself, *how the hell are they going to get me out of here? There's no way I can move!* I closed my eyes, took a deep breath, placed my right leg over the side of the birth tub, and lifted my left leg to a ninety-degree angle. On the next contraction, I was going to push hard and deep. No longer would I care about tearing. I would push until my son was out.

I felt the contraction coming, and I pushed with my eyes closed, moaning and spreading my legs as far as I could. I could hear Claudette get up, move around to the front of the tub to see between my legs, and heard her say, "Yup."

Laura said to me, "There you go, mama, you got this. You are strong and fierce. Do it. Don't stop."

I got ready to push again, but Jason wasn't with me. He was in the kitchen on the phone. Claudette told him to get off the stupid phone and watch his son be born.

Jason replied to her, "But I can't hang up on Nana!"

I said "Jason, tell Nana I love her and we will call her when this is over. Get your ass over here now."

Jason hung up and came over to my right side and grabbed my hand. On the next contraction, I pushed hard and long. I kept breathing so I could keep pushing.

Jason said, "There's his head, Selena. You got it!"

Pretty sure I let out a yell. I tried to push again.

One of the midwives said, "Selena, don't push if you're not having a contraction."

All I could picture was Blaine's head sticking halfway out and then going back inside and me having to go through this all over again. Suddenly, the wave came over me, the next contraction, push! His head was out! Everyone was cheering, even Jason. It was so awesome, and I had a burst of energy. Last contraction, *boom*! Out came Blaine, and I threw my head back.

When I lifted my head, I could see Claudette holding Blaine up in the air. The cord was wrapped around him several times, neck and body. In the blink of an eye, Laura and Claudette got him unwrapped and tossed him on my chest. No vernix! I looked down at him and kept telling him I loved him. The midwives were rubbing him with receiving blankets, sucking his throat, and cleaning him while he was on me, then he cried out. The midwives cheered and told him to keep on crying. I was in total shock. I looked over to find Jason who was in the kitchen, bent over the counter, his shirt up over his eyes, crying. I looked back at Blaine. Holy crap, I did it. *We* did it. My son was in my arms, and he was doing great. My midwives kept telling me to keep holding him up, hold him up out of the water; he was in too far. I didn't think I had enough left in me to hold my son. He wasn't breast crawling either, he was just staring at me. I wanted Jason to take the baby. I didn't want to drop him in the water, but I couldn't verbalize that. Jason knelt down, hugged me, and kissed me on top of my head.

Jason whispered, "You did it babe, you did it."

I felt so proud. Having my husband acknowledge everything I had gone through to carry our child and birth him safely at home like I wanted meant so much to me.

I closed my eyes, put my hand on his neck, and I could feel our son against my chest. There are no words to describe this feeling. Laura took a great photo of the moment. Then Claudette came around to see Blaine and ask me how I was doing. You would think I would have become emotional earlier, but no. Once I saw Claudette, all the emotion came out. She took us under her wing, taught us about the birth process, and recommended natural herbs and remedies that helped keep me strong through labor.

I'll never forget when Claudette told me, "You can do anything for sixty seconds, remember that."

Claudette told me how proud she was of me. Proud that I overcame all the negativity to have the birth I wanted, but mostly that I powered through and brought my son safely earth-side. Claudette also explained to me that Blaine had come down the birth canal with his arm up and bent over his face, causing me pain and making it difficult to get him under my bone. She also concluded that at some point he went breech, which is why he was so wrapped up in his cord.

"The next baby won't be this difficult, it'll be much easier for you," she said.

"Nope. Nope. Nope," was all I could mutter!

Suddenly I felt almost like an itching or a burning in my vaginal area. I shifted my bottom and told the midwives, "something feels funny." I pushed. Out came my placenta in one piece. Laura said, "Oh, sh*t!"

She grabbed my placenta and went to put it in the bowl. Somehow, the placenta dropped on my legs; blood was everywhere. Normally I would vomit. I don't do blood, and I sure as hell didn't want to see my placenta. She picked it up in the bowl, and there we were: Mommy, Blaine and the placenta floating around in the birth tub.

The cord stopped pulsing around thirty minutes after I had the baby. It was time to cut the cord. I didn't have the stomach for that, so Claudette helped Jason cut the cord while I was still in the tub. After that, it was time for me to get out and go on the couch. I felt great. I laid on the couch with Blaine, trying to get him to latch on and FaceTiming with my doula and sister-in-law, Caitlin. My Siamese cat, Prince, jumped up on the couch to check everything out, too!

The midwives started to clean up and make food. I didn't want anything, just a coke! Claudette made me a peanut butter and jelly sandwich, got me a coke, and a water. I relaxed on the couch for a few more minutes. I was hot and tired. Jason took Blaine and did skin to skin with him, and I glanced over to see my husband and the baby on the stairs, taking photos, Jason cooing at the babe. I giggled. My husband was the happiest I had ever seen him. At this point, I told Laura and Claudette I wanted to go upstairs. Different fluids were leaking from my body, and I knew I needed a different position. They weren't quite sure that I was going to be able to climb the steep stairs to our bedroom, but I felt fine and wanted to be closer to the bathroom and in the bed.

So up we went, Laura helping me up while Claudette made the most awesome pillow fort I have ever seen on my bed. Jason was standing in the corner, snuggling Blaine. Laura may have brought the computer upstairs as well so Caitlin could stay with us. I'm pretty sure my brother was on, as well. I went to the bathroom. That was ouch. Small needle prick feeling sensation. Laura made me a peri wash rinse with warm water and something else to help me heal, and showed me how to use it and clean up. I put on my granny panties and a big pad. So sexy. I walked back to bed and got all propped up. We noticed I had some blood on my ankles from when I was leaking downstairs; Laura actually washed my feet and ankles. Our midwives' care was amazing.

Then it was time to do my checkup. Claudette wanted to make sure I didn't tear.

I asked her, "I can decline stitches, right?"

She replied, "You are such a pain in the ass, but yes, you can."

After a good check and double check, she told me I didn't tear. Hallelujah! Minor "skid marks" and one little nick, that was it. Phew. All that Vitamin C worked! After that, we did Blaine's checkup. We took guesses before we weighed and measured him. He ended up being seven pounds, six and a half ounces and twenty-one inches, our long and lanky babe! Daddy did the honors of putting his first diaper on him and his first onesie, Batman.

Shortly after, my incredible midwives said goodbye. We exchanged love and gratitude. These women had become an essential part of my life and my family's life. It was sad having them leave. They closed the door behind them, and Jason crawled in bed with me and Blaine. There we were: the Three Musketeers. Ready to begin our lives together as one.

Chapter 6

Home Birth after Cesarean Section? Yes, You Can!

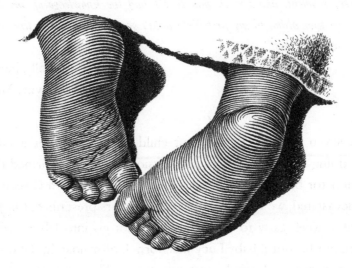

Molly's Home Birth
after a Cesarean

○ ○ ○ ○ ○ ○ ○ ○ • • • • • ○ • ○ ○ ○ ◦

"Although it was a long (almost forty-three-hour) labor, I wouldn't change one thing! I loved every moment, and I'm so glad that I had the knowledge of my midwives reminding me that although my first birth didn't go as planned, this time would be different; it certainly was!"

—Molly, hair stylist
Bellevue, Michigan

At thirty-seven weeks with our first child, Lucy, and after a failed attempt at doing an External Cephalic Version, we were informed that the only option for birthing our Frank breech little girl was a C-section. Although devastated, we went with what the doctors prescribed. On January 3rd, 2009, a week early to ensure I would not go into labor before the C-section, our beautiful baby Lucy was born. Unfortunately, the operation and after-care was cold, sterile, and impersonal. The experience turned us off to hospital births.

Over the course of the next few years, we had many birth discussions with a midwife, Kim Woodard-Osterholzer, that went to our church. Kim and her daughter, Hannah Woodard-Simmons (also an amazing midwife), helped us prepare and plan for our home birth. Both midwives were there for us every step of the way.

Collectively, we decided that when I did get pregnant, it would be wise to receive dual care in case anything went south. We found an obstetrician (OB) we felt comfortable working with, and I felt deeply that the Lord's protective hand was all over the whole pregnancy and birth. With having an OB, the biggest thing was making sure my scar tissue and placenta were doing what they needed to do to make sure the birth would be successful. We let him know from the beginning that we planned on a home birth, which he wasn't one hundred percent on board with, and saw him just as often as if we were going to have him in the hospital. As we approached my estimated due date of October 9th, 2015, the OB seemed a little apprehensive here and there (especially as we passed my due date by a few weeks), but I was prepared and determined! We had finished our birthing class, and I felt like I could do anything. Little did I know I was going to be waiting a bit longer than we thought to welcome our handsome little guy.

At 3:00 a.m. on October 29th, I awoke to the feeling of peeing my bed. Faster than I'd moved in weeks, I jumped out of bed to find that my water had broken! My husband quickly woke up, helped me into the shower while I experienced my very first contraction, and immediately called our midwife, Hannah. Hannah told us to get ready and to set up like we'd discussed. She also wanted us to time the contractions when they started getting closer together and to call when they were five minutes apart. We decided Grandma's was the best place to be for Miss Lucy and then spent most of the day doing chores and trying to stay busy with contractions between five and fifteen minutes apart. Around midafternoon, the contractions quickened and Hannah and her apprentice, Heather, came out.

After Hannah and Heather set up and did my first BP check and listened for our little guy's heart, they hung out and we chatted for a bit between contractions. They helped me through the tough ones with Gordy by my side, but mostly they let him and I be just be while still being there for support when needed. I labored pretty steadily the rest of the evening and into the early morning using my exercise ball and walking around a lot of the time.

On the second day of being in labor at around 5:30 a.m., Hannah decided it would be best to check me for progress since it had been more than twenty-four hours since my water broke. I was only at a 4, and my contractions had slowed back down to five to ten minutes apart. The midwives decided it was a good opportunity for them to go home to get cleaned up and rest while we went on a breakfast date together. I had an appointment with my chiropractor already scheduled for that morning, so Hannah advised that I keep it and get adjusted. After the chiropractor appointment, we went to breakfast (all the while still having regular contractions). Hannah had suggested a walk, so we did that while doing a little grocery shopping.

I came home exhausted, and immediately took a nap. I woke up to steady and strong contractions (about one minute long and two minutes apart). Hannah and Heather came back and we continued with super steady contractions. Hannah checked me again when I said I was really feeling pushy at about 8:30 that evening. She found that I was only at a nine and that I was a little inflamed. She had me lay on my side and try to relax for a half an hour. I took two different dissolving homeopathic tablets, Arnica and Gelsemium, to help calm and soothe my bothered and swollen cervix during that half hour. Still having regular and hard contractions, I started to feel as though I was peeing the bed (again!). Finally, when my time was almost up, I said I just had to get to the bathroom asap!

This was when I realized, as I sat down to find an intense gush of water coming out of me, why they call it your waters breaking and why my labor had taken so long. My first layer of the amniotic sac broke in bed the morning before, but the second layer breaking was where the real fun began. I suddenly felt that hot nauseous feeling rushing over my whole body, and I knew right then and there what the difference between labor and "active labor" was. Immediately I had the urge to push, and a few contractions later, with the help of my hubby, I'd gotten myself back to the bedroom where all was set up and ready. Heather came in as I was on my hands and knees on the bed, wanting to check the baby's heart rate with the Doppler. I refused and informed her she would be able to check it in a minute because he'd be out soon!

I gave one good solid push up on the bed, and Hannah knew quickly that position wasn't going to be the best for me. She asked me if I could quickly and carefully get off the bed and come down to the birthing stool. I did, and another contraction came almost immediately. With another push, he crowned. I asked to see and feel what was going on down there. As soon as I touched him, a final push rushed in and out came our beautiful boy. He slid first into my Love's hands, then Hannah's, then my husband's again! My husband passed our baby to me. We quickly and carefully moved to the bed where I held him and we looked him over and cried together. He was just so perfect. Hannah and Heather had already cleaned up the floor area and asked if I could give one last push for the afterbirth. I easily did. After taking the yucky sheets and drop cloth, she placed the placenta still attached to and giving nourishment to my boy in a bag next to me while I nursed him for the first time. Then, after a few hours she brought us some food, clamped the umbilical cord, and let Gordy cut it (which he did with his father's buck knife) and then did the placenta and baby exam right there in bed with us.

Although it was a long (almost forty-three hour) labor, I wouldn't change one thing! I loved every moment, and I'm so glad that I had the knowledge of my midwives reminding me that although my first birth didn't go as planned, this time would be different; it certainly was!

A Home Birth after
Two Cesarean Sections

○ ○ ○ ○ ○ ○ ○ ○ • • • • • • • ○ (○

"My husband and I both agree that there's a place where the hospital and intervention is great; that was the case with our first baby's birth. But if all is going normally, we both agreed a midwife's care is more intimate and individualized, and we would prefer to just stay in the comfort and calm of our own home surrounded by our other children."

—L. Baker, mother and artist

Georgia

A little background: my husband Michael and I had our first daughter in the Summer of 2007. We planned for an un-medicated hospital delivery with a midwife, but at twenty weeks an issue with our daughter's neck was found. Our plan was changed to a scary, but necessary, C-section at thirty-eight weeks under general anesthesia with a special procedure and NICU time. All went as well as we could have hoped and we were able to go home sooner than expected. Then, we got the shock of our lives and found out we were expecting again. Our second baby's due date was the same as our first baby's, just a year later. We wanted to VBAC (vaginal birth after Cesarean), but our doctor wasn't comfortable with the closeness of our pregnancies or the closeness of our due date to his scheduled vacation. So, in the summer of 2008, at thirty-eight weeks two days, we had a "normal" scheduled repeat C-section while "Hey Jude" played on the loudspeaker.

During the surgery, my doctor noted that I had almost no scar tissue and probably could have VBAC-ed after all. Those words sent me to search out as much information as I could about VBAC before we had our third child. In that search, I found ICAN, the International Cesarean Awareness Network, and my local chapter, ICAN of Atlanta. This group of ladies told me about a doctor, Dr. T., who trusted women's bodies and had not only attended VBACS, but VBAC2Cs, and VBAC3Cs, and VBACS for multiples.

We found out we were expecting our third child, E, in early 2010 and asked our OB who delivered our first two children about VBAC2C. He was not supportive at first. When we mentioned wanting a second opinion, he changed his tone, but said if I didn't go into labor by forty weeks, a VBAC wasn't going to happen. We switched care to Dr. T., and at forty weeks and three days had our third baby so quickly that Dr. T. missed the birth! It was an amazing experience, and I was so thankful for his care. But as we sat with our doula and the sun set over Atlanta, we all seemed to have the same sentiment: the day was wonderful, but it would have been even more special if we would have stayed home to have the birth.

And that brings us to baby number four, Katarina. It happened again.

As I ate a pita sandwich of mozzarella, ranch dressing, and barbecue sauce, Michael exclaimed, "You're pregnant!"

"No, I can't be. This is just a nursing mom craving."

Less than an hour later we were sure he was right. Baby number four was expected to arrive just thirteen months after baby number three. From the start, we felt this baby needed a name that started with K, all our favorite names did, so we called the baby K.

I contacted my doula, Talitha, who attended the birth of our third child, and we went back to Dr. T. to confirm. Yep, pregnant again. But where my OB with my first two had been scared of my births being so close together, Dr. T. seemed unfazed. Just like with E's pregnancy, he was great, but something was weighing on us.

With E's birth, we labored so well at home before going to the hospital, and then with our doctor missing it, it just felt like more confirmation that we should have stayed home. We talked with our doula about our feelings, and she helped us research local home birth midwives with VBAC experience.

At the time, there were three main VBAC supportive midwives near Atlanta. Of the three, one stood out. Her name was Brenda, and she'd recently moved to the area. She had a medical background, but was a traditional midwife, soon to finish her CPM certification. She was Christian, which was important to us, and had attended home births after multiple Cesareans (HBAMCs) before. While planning interviews, we asked Talitha to reach out to all our perspective midwives for us. We got a call back that the other two midwives we were looking at were under backup doctors who were not VBAC supportive.

I'll admit this fact was scary. Despite all the research we'd done assuring us home birth was a safe option, we found ourselves wondering if this was the path we were meant to be on. At almost 9:00 p.m. Michael and I prayed and said that if we were meant to have a home birth that Brenda would be our provider. If she was not open to working with us, we would take it as a sign that this wasn't meant to be and continue on the path to another hospital delivery. As we said "amen," my cell phone rang. It was Brenda. After speaking with her, I felt working with Brenda was truly meant to be. Brenda even mentioned how she prayed about which clients she was meant to take on before committing, and I felt even more confident that a home birth with Brenda as our midwife was the right choice for our family. After our final twenty-eight week OB appointment we switched providers and started down the journey to HBA2C.

Care with our midwife was intimate and comfortable. It was the perfect blend of medical and natural, all while my two toddlers and baby played nearby. In the final week before K's birth, I began feeling exhausted. This was significantly different to the energy boost I had for weeks at the end of my pregnancy with E. Michael was awesome about helping me get in some extra rest. He said I should listen to my body and joked that my body was probably storing up energy for the work ahead.

I had a sudden burst of energy the day before my due date. We went to the same restaurant we had dinner at the night before E's arrival. Although I didn't expect to go into labor, I hoped it might happen that way again. The next day, my estimated due date, I woke up at 2:00 a.m. with pink discharge. I thought this might be the start of labor since this was how E's birth began. I had a few contractions that were three to five minutes apart, but not consistent in duration. I had a small glass of wine and a bath, since this helped me relax with E. Instead of just relaxing me, while everything continued, the contractions stopped completely. At 4:00 a.m., feeling frustrated and a bit disappointed, I headed back to bed.

Thanks to the early morning excitement, we slept in a bit. I woke up later and went to the bathroom: there was more mucous plug with pink on the paper. When E took her afternoon nap, I laid down with her and got some extra rest. I woke up to more discharge, this time with dark red in it.

My mother-in-law (who we call Ibu) came over a bit before 5:00 p.m. for a visit and to help prepare food for our "babymoon." We played with the kids, and Ibu spent lots of time in the kitchen cooking and freezing food. Ibu was convinced I was going into labor that day; she claimed she was being affected by my hormones. However, other than the mucous plug (which I had already begun losing weeks before) I felt great and didn't see labor coming on any time soon.

We all stayed up late that night. Ibu decided to stay past when hubby and I went to bed, because she wanted to make sure all the cooking was done. E was awake a little longer wanting to play with Ibu, but she went to bed for the first time in her own crib for the entire night. Thank goodness too, as I woke up around 2:00 a.m. with contractions. Michael got up with me and we spoke with Ibu. The contractions were pretty strong, but I doubted they were real since the previous day's fake out. During each contraction, it felt best to lean over the counters in the kitchen and move my legs back and forth like I was doing lunges.

Though skeptical, Ibu had been supportive of our home birth plans. However, she was very clear she wouldn't be there for the birth. Ibu joked about leaving right then. But because we'd been up late and Michael was tired, we decided it'd be nice if she stayed just in case things picked up and became "real" so Michael could go back to bed. Ibu compared the way I was working out the contractions to how she'd been at the beginning of her labor with her third child. She thought this was the real thing for sure, but I didn't.

I decided to take a bath (again) and figured things would stop or at least calm down for us to go back to bed. Contractions were all about three minutes apart and only thirty to forty-five seconds in length; much easier than E's, so I figured I still had plenty of time. As I soaked in the tub, I continued comparing this birth to my last. I kept expecting everything to progress on the same schedule, in the same way as before, despite the many women who'd told me that every birth is different. I didn't get it. Little did I know the surprise I was in for.

The bath didn't help with the contractions; in fact, things seemed to be accelerating instead of staying consistent like last time. I kept trying to shift positions and relax, but I couldn't even find comfort sitting down. I got out of the bath around 3:30 a.m. and went to talk with Ibu. I lamented that it didn't hurt this much last time. She assured me it did, although maybe not so soon or I'd forgotten. I told her this was different.

I was really worried about waking Michael up because he definitely hadn't gotten enough sleep, and I knew he'd probably need it "if this was real" (still had the denial going despite everything). I worked through the contractions by walking around and talking with Ibu.

Now, honestly, I never in a million years imagined I would want my mother-in-law with me during labor, any more than she thought she would want to be there, but she was who I needed. She was the right mix of support, reality check, humor, sarcasm, and comfort. She also seemed to know the hip squeeze comfort maneuver like a pro. I am still in shock how well it worked out.

I had planned to call my mom in early labor to come watch the kids, but since they were asleep and my mom is not a night owl, I knew I'd be more worried about her driving to us so early in the morning and about her reaction to seeing me in pain than it would be worth at that point. Ibu's tough love seemed to just work, and she said she would stay as long as we wanted or needed, so we decided to keep working together, just the two of us.

Around 5:00 a.m. things were getting much more intense. I told Ibu how bad I felt to wake Michael and our midwife that early, but that the way the pains were going, I felt I needed to call my midwife, Brenda. I also told Ibu how crazy it was to imagine calling so soon because last time, at this stage, I still had twelve hours before delivery. Ibu reminded me it was Brenda's job to come, and if it wasn't the real thing (though she thought it was), Brenda would understand. I gave in and called. Brenda asked me about how quickly I had progressed last time. I said I did progress quickly toward the end, but this birth felt different. I was, however, still convinced that both births would play out the same way.

Ibu woke Michael up, and although I couldn't stop apologizing for his lack of sleep, I was very happy he was there. He never complained about the lack of sleep. Instead, he jumped into birth mode. We walked through the contractions, and I found significant relief by leaning against a living room wall under a picture of my first three children while doing lunges. Michael also did hip squeezes on me and Ibu rubbed my lower back between contractions. This was similar to the motions/massage that my doula Talitha did a lot further on during E's birth.

Michael inflated the birth tub (though we didn't fill it with any water) and covered the floor in tablecloths turned upside down (so the felt side was up to prevent sliding) and shower curtain liners. Not too long after I first called Brenda, I decided I needed to call again. I told her things had picked up a lot, and I was getting a little nervous at how quickly labor was progressing without our midwife there. Michael called my doula, Talitha, at 5:47 a.m. Talitha asked Michael if we wanted her to head over.

I responded, "If she wants to be here for the delivery, she'd better." She said she'd be leaving shortly.

The contractions continued to pick up as we waited for everyone to arrive. I wasn't hungry, but a little tired, and knew I needed to keep hydrated. I tried the coconut water all my friends had recommended and raved about. The sweetness was overwhelming, though, and I switched to water and lemon Gatorade between contractions.

Though my senses seemed to be heightened during pregnancy, it was worse during labor. My taste buds and sense of smell were even more sensitive. I started feeling a little nauseous because of this, though thankfully didn't get sick.

Our midwife, Brenda, arrived around 5:30 a.m., despite how much I'd researched and planned for home birth, I was still impressed by how extensive her birth kit and tools were. My living room seemed to quickly fill with precautionary devices and items for baby care and after delivery. Even through the very intense contractions, I noticed and felt reassured that in the case of an emergency, we were in good hands.

The contractions were getting more intense and closer together; my water was starting to leak a little during each contraction. Brenda took K's heart rate. It was in the 140s. Brenda mentioned she doubted we'd have time to fill the birth tub up. I hadn't planned to deliver in the water because I thought it might dull the feeling of touching the baby's head and catching her myself so I wasn't upset about this news. I was still in denial about being in labor. Brenda asked to check me, and I consented mainly because I wanted to know if this was the real thing. Lying on the floor between contractions was not easy. I was eight and a half centimeters, almost complete, and she reassured me this wasn't going to stop anytime soon.

Talitha, our doula, arrived not too long after Brenda. Ibu got some tea cozy rice pads we had and placed them on my back and then rotated coming in the living room to help where she could and running back in the kitchen to cook more. I moved from my wall lunges to kneeling over my peanut ball and next to our loveseat on the floor. Talitha took over putting pressure on my mid-back. Michael kept up hip squeezes, letting me lean on him, and being amazing in his labor dad/husband mode. It impressed me how he stepped up during E's birth, but during K's birth, he was even more amazing.

At one point our eldest child woke up, and Ibu helped her back to sleep by encouraging her to dream of a new sister who was a baby princess. Shockingly, she went back to sleep quickly. The timing of events worked out really well as everything was happening while the kids were asleep. I had told Michael before that I thought the time I was most relaxed was when they were all in bed, and I'm glad it worked out that way.

Brenda's midwife apprentice, Jen, arrived shortly after Talitha. Along with assisting Brenda, she took pictures for us, as well. I felt comforted and supported by her presence, but never interrupted by it. I definitely see her as being a great midwife in the future.

Around 6:45 a.m., my water was leaking more with each contraction, and I began occasionally pushing. I felt significant pressure and I felt like I was pushing, but my head started getting in my body's way. I felt I was doing everything wrong and started focusing on everyone around me. Every time someone whispered, even though it didn't have anything to do with me directly, I thought they were criticizing me by whispering what I was doing wrong.

I was complete, but K was still pretty high. Everyone kept telling me I needed to bring her down, but I didn't know how to get that done. Hold my breath, don't hold my breath, growl, don't let your voice go too high, low tones . . . no one was directing me, but my own worries and stage fright (from my first delivery) were in full force. I asked for everyone to pray for me. Brenda said a wonderful prayer aloud which helped me focus a little more, but I was still fighting myself.

This is when the worries and doubts really came, and I started working things out in my head. This wasn't working: the position, the pushing, the focus, everything was wrong. The only pain relief I asked for was Tylenol, in jest, but I didn't want pain relief; I wanted my baby. I thought about alternatives. I did have choices. In a hospital, ineffective long-term pushing would most likely end in C-section, though maybe in a best-case scenario I would only get vacuum or forceps. Yes, the baby would be out, but I would be forced to endure weeks of physical pain and years of mental and emotional distress knowing I could have birthed at home, if I hadn't got in my own way. I started my own mini-mantra saying, "I can do this" and "I am doing this" over and over.

The pressure was building, and I tried to focus more intently. I pushed harder and actually pooped a bit. Despite any worries prior to birth, I felt zero embarrassment at having pooped; this at least proved I was doing something right! I pushed again, and the rest of my water gushed out. Talitha reminded me that during E's labor, she was born soon after my waters broke. It was at this moment that I finally realized and truly accepted that this is not E's birth.

Obviously, the same position wasn't working. I decided to put aside any worries about delivering in water and asked to get in the bath tub. Someone suggested I try a couple contractions on the toilet. This actually felt really good. With more pressure came more bowel movements; this made being on the toilet extra convenient. I knew I didn't want to give birth on the toilet, but I allowed myself to relax a little. The contractions seemed to get a little more manageable now that I was in the bathroom with just Michael. I'm not sure if they were actually physically easier or just mentally easier. I worried that easier contractions were a bad sign, but I pushed the thought from my mind. I choose to believe that God was watching over us, everything was okay, and we just needed to figure out how to work through this moment in K's birth.

Someone turned the lights off, only allowing the sun's light to shine through the edge of the blinds. Brenda checked me and K's heart rate, but then stayed outside the door encouraging Michael to stay in with me; just the two, soon to be three, of us. Eventually, we moved to the bathtub. Being in the tub felt great, but the water didn't dull all the sensations. It did, however, allow me to mentally work through that stage of labor.

I should note that our rental house is older, and the tub is small. It has two glass sliding doors which can only be open one at a time. One would think this small tub wouldn't be conducive to birthing, but when we were in the living room and I had several sets of hands on my back and many comforting faces to look at, I was getting too caught up in the feeling that we had an audience. I felt safer and more relaxed with just Michael holding my hand in the dark of the bathroom with the sun peeking through the small window. This privacy and intimacy is something I know I wouldn't have been able to have in a hospital.

I balanced my forearms on the sides of the tub and used the leverage to squat in the water. I was still contracting and losing the mucous plug. I started feeling around to apply counterpressure. I pressed around the skin on the various sides of my vulva. I could feel where K was by way of pressure. Her head was more toward my back, putting pressure on my bottom. We believe she may have been posterior, and the reason she took longer to descend, despite my being complete, was her turning through all this, combined with her bigger size.

I started visualizing and figuring out where she was and where I needed her to be. I pressed around the edge of my vulva when pushing. I shifted from squat to a kind of side lie and moved back and forth. I talked to K during all this. I would say, "Okay I need you to move this way, you're too far back. I'll tilt this and you shift here. Good. Now you need to move down." It might sound crazy, but it worked! I felt a little inside to see if what I felt was actual progress and was surprised by a rubbery feeling squished ball with what felt like wet hair on it. I yelled, "Brenda I feel something! Something is happening!"

Brenda quickly came in asking Michael, "She thinks she feels the head?"

I responded, "Well, it's not me, for sure."

Soon there was no doubting that K's head was about to be born. Brenda mentioned how I probably needed to change to a position for pushing since I was in a kind of can opener pose (one leg up, one down awkwardly in our small bathtub). I couldn't imagine sitting or lying back as much, but I tried shifting to a squat for the next push then laying back for the next; it worked. K was definitely coming now. Once again, compared to E's birth, when I pushed once and her head partially came out, K was determined to prove to me that this was not her sister's birth.

K was coming out much more slowly. I could feel everything (my worries about the water dulling things were null). I felt her slowly crowning and felt the ring of fire coming, as well (this definitely was more pronounced than during E's birth). I felt my skin stretching with each centimeter as she moved further out.

With one push, K's head slowly emerged and the contraction stopped. Suddenly, I was sitting there waiting with her head out.

Michael told me, "You're doing it, hun! She's right there!"

My response was, "No, sh*t."

Not my finest moment, but I'm not sure if anyone could've missed that there was a baby coming out of me at this point. He reached down to feel her head and help guide her out. Brenda checked her heart rate again and the cord to make sure it wasn't around K's neck. It was on her upper torso, and when she told me, I reached down and gently pulled it off.

All was truly perfect. Jen and Talitha were present and reassuring. Jen is very tall and, thankfully, she was able to get some pictures from above the bath. I felt as though this birth was just Michael and me bringing this baby into the world together, just as she was created by the two of us.

It felt like forever as I waited for another contraction to push again.

I yelled toward Brenda and Michael, "Just pull her out! I want another contraction!"

An hour beforehand I never could've imagined such a request. I can now understand how some women might enjoy pushing more than the first stage . . . maybe.

Michael continued supporting me through everything. At 8:25 a.m., in one of the most beautiful moments of my life, and of my husband's and my relationship, K turned, slid out, and was born with my hands under her arms and her daddy's hands first on her head, then moving down to help lift her bottom and feet up onto me. We brought our baby Katarina onto my chest together.

I could tell she was beautiful from the start. I did double check to make sure she was still a she. I was surprised at how much dark blonde curly hair she had. At some point during the pushing stage, the lights had been turned back on. K's forehead was a little purple from pushing, but she quickly pinked up. Her Apgar score was 9/9. She had some congestion, which Brenda suctioned out. Everyone kept saying how big and healthy she was, but she seemed tiny to me.

K lay contently on my chest with a few little "mews." She kept exploring with her tiny long fingers and actually grasped my cross necklace for a bit. This moment meant a lot to me because this necklace was worn by my great grandmother, who is my namesake, when she had my grandmother, my mother when she had me, my husband when I had our first two babies, (because I wasn't allowed any jewelry), and by me during E's birth last year. It was a reminder of how far my family and I have been in our birth journeys and how much God has blessed us.

Afterward we called my mom to tell her there was someone she needed to meet. We stayed in the bath until the cord stopped pulsing, and then Michael cut it. We had to wait for the placenta, and Brenda had to help a little in getting it to pass. We believe I had a succenturiate placenta, meaning there's an extra lobe on the side of it which was retained. This didn't affect K's growth. The only impact was the way the placenta came out. I didn't worry even with this slight complication since we were in the best of hands under Brenda's care. It's amazing to me how much can be done in the home and all the precautions that are taken. When people think about home birth I don't think they realize the level of care being given. And Brenda in particular was truly the best midwife for our family.

After the placenta passed, the tub was prepared for an herbal sitz bath. We all moved to the bedroom with Brenda while the rest of our support crew cleaned up the living room and bathroom.

Ibu and Michael woke up the kids so they could meet their new sister, Katarina. Our eldest remembered the baby princess from her dreams and kept saying, "K's so pretty. I love her." Our son knew this baby was K, but kept asking how she got out of Mommy's belly. And E was a little overwhelmed since she didn't recognize all the new faces of our birth team, but she was very happy to check out her new baby sis. She surprised us by taking a hat to try and dress her baby sis (when normally she takes other people's clothes just to put on herself).

Brenda completed the newborn exam and was very patient with excited siblings trying to help. Katarina's stats were nine pounds six ounces and twenty-two inches long, our biggest baby to date. Afterward, I felt blissful, though a bit more tired than after E's birth, which could just be attributed to one more child, not much sleep, or no hospital mommy down time. But everything went exactly how it was supposed to. I am so very thankful for my midwives' and doula's care, my husband's strength and comfort, and the surprise aid of my mother-in-law.

I think back to how our birth progressed. In a hospital, had I gone through the same thing, I am very doubtful most providers would have shown me the same patience or allowed my husband and I to go aside, with me in the water, and the lights off. That space was exactly what Katarina and I truly needed. I am thankful we were led down the home birth path; it was the best birth option for us, our baby, and our family.

Emily's Beautiful Home Birth

○ ○ ○ ○ ○ ○ ○ ○ ○ ○ ○ ○ ○ ○ (○

"From the very beginning of my third pregnancy, I knew I wanted to have a home birth after my successful, all natural vaginal birth after Cesarean section (VBAC) in the hospital. However, we were devastated when we lost our daughter at seventeen weeks of pregnancy. When I became pregnant one year later with our son, I knew I still wanted to fulfill my desire to have a home birth. I believed I could do it, and I wanted to be comfortable in familiar surroundings."

—Emily, lactation professional and stay-at-home mom
Marietta, Georgia

Our home birth happened to take place at our guest house, which is a vacation rental home. We now rent our guest house out to other expectant moms who wish to have a home birth experience, but for whatever reason, don't want to or cannot do it at their own homes. I'm glad we can support other home birth families with alternative options.

At thirty-eight weeks and four days, I began having strong contractions, but nothing consistent. I started listening to my "Come Out, Baby" Hypnobabies track at 12:00 p.m., and it put me right to sleep. I woke up two hours later with real contractions. Although they were strong, the contractions were still fairly irregular. I tried resting, but the twinges kept me half awake. Later that evening, around 9:00 p.m., I had my first bloody show. For me, that is a guarantee of real labor. I called my parents who were flying down for the birth, and texted my midwives, Paige and Rachel, and my photographer, Vania, to give them a heads-up that labor was beginning. Ian and I headed over to the birth house to set everything up. Ian had a momentary moment of panic: we were all alone, and I was in labor. I had to focus on keeping myself calm, as I knew that stress could stall my labor. I reminded him that I tended to have long labors, and I wouldn't be delivering for quite a while, so he did not need to worry about catching a baby on his own. Fortunately, he returned to center fairly quickly, and we finished getting our space ready. We prepared the bed, laid down our protective floor coverings, and set up the birthing space in the master bathroom garden tub.

Contractions picked up in duration, regularity, and intensity about 2:00 a.m. I called my birth team soon after and everyone arrived around 3:30 a.m. we filled the garden tub and I got in. I was having intense, no joke, back labor. We already knew baby was posterior, despite having tried optimal positioning and chiropractic adjustments to encourage him to flip over in the last few weeks. I was really hopeful he would flip during labor like the majority of babies do, as per the Spinning Babies website. No luck!

I got out of the tub once around 7:00 a.m. to change things up. I started feeling nauseous and vomited (first time that's happened in any of my labors). I decided to labor on the bed with a peanut ball between my knees to help keep my pelvis open and also to encourage baby to get into proper position. At this point I asked Paige to check me for the first time, not expecting to be that far dilated as my labors tend to go marathon-long. To my surprise, I was eight and a half centimeters dilated! My back labor was so much more intense on the bed, and no amount of back massage was helping. I wanted back in the tub immediately. The hot water was a big relief for a few minutes, and then I really started to feel baby move through the bones of my pelvis. I began to grunt-push involuntarily through the peak of each contraction. Around 8:00 a.m. I started to actively push through each contraction. I pushed leaning back against the tub, then I moved to a reclined-squat with my feet braced against the front of the tub and my back to the back of the tub. I could start to feel the burn of baby's head crowning, but I just couldn't get the leverage I needed to push him out. I gave another big push and my bag of water broke.

Paige and Rachel suggested that I try getting on my hands and knees to push, but I was in so much discomfort that I didn't want to move. Plus, baby was twisting (trying to flip over?) during the crowning, and it was incredibly painful. Finally, my husband insisted I try turning, and he grabbed my arms and helped me get on my knees in the water: best thing ever! I believe that my pelvis was able to widen to allow easier passage.

I pushed hard with the next contraction and felt his head pop out. Paige unwrapped some cord from around his neck. I waited for the next contraction. At 10:04 a.m., I gave another strong push, and his whole body was born. Paige passed him through my legs, and I brought him up and out of the water. It was amazing!

From this point, it was a little dicey. While Graham had handled the entire labor beautifully with his heart rate in the 140s, he came out totally blue, limp and quiet with Apgars of 6 at one minute. Rachel urgently requested everyone to help me out of the tub. The oxygen was grabbed and administered. Suctioning began while we rubbed and talked to Graham. In hindsight, this probably would have had me totally freaking out, but in the moment, I wasn't worried. Rachel and Paige were calm and confident during his resuscitation. At five minutes his Apgars were 9. It could have happened anywhere. It was most likely the combination of him being large, the cord being wrapped around his neck, and his posterior positioning that caused the cord to compress enough to make him pass out. I am grateful that we had a skilled birth team who knew exactly what to do, and quickly.

We retreated to the bed while I waited to deliver the placenta, which came about thirty minutes later. I received a prophylactic injection of Pitocin as we had previously discussed to help prevent another postpartum hemorrhage. Paige asked me to give a little push; just that little bit of pressure caused the placenta and tons of fluid to come flying out! She said she had never seen anyone deliver a placenta like that, and we all laughed. After about forty-five minutes I cut the cord myself, and an embroidered cord tie with a small race car design was used to tie off the umbilical cord. Graham was the rosiest baby I'd ever seen due to delayed cord clamping, and he stayed like that for many weeks.

After a few hours, Graham was examined by Paige, weighed and measured. He was ten pounds and twenty-two and a quarter inches long. He was huge! Despite his size and mal-positioning, Graham's labor was the shortest labor of my three at *only* eighteen hours. Ian's parents arrived with our two girls to meet their brother just after Graham's birth, and everyone was all smiles and excitement. My mother and father arrived shortly after, though my mom was heartbroken that she missed his birth by only a short window of time. I was so happy to see my mom as she is an amazing postpartum doula (as well as a skilled birth attendant and herself a home birther); I was in wonderful hands for the next two weeks.

We spent the first blissful days in bed, skin-to-skin with my newborn, and getting breastfeeding well-established. As a lactation educator and counselor, I know how important the early days are for breastfeeding. We took Graham for his first pediatrician appointment two days later for his hearing check and expanded newborn genetic screening from hunter-shope.org. Our pediatrician is supportive of home birth and made us feel so comfortable. Our dedicated birth team was wonderful before, during, and after our home birth, and I would do it again in a heartbeat!

Chapter 7

All in Good Time

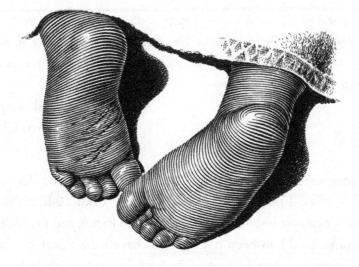

Milli from the Positive
Birth Movement

○ ○ ○ ○ ○ ○ ○ ○ ○ ○ ○ ○ ○ ○ ○ ○ ○ ◦ ◦ ◦

"George ripped off his clothes and jumped in the water to be closer to us, and Bess was helped out of her pajamas so she could do the same. It was an incredible moment—the four of us—a woman empowered and a family made new, in the very healing waters."

—Milli, writer and campaigner
United Kingdom

It was during my first pregnancy that I was introduced to the idea of water birth. Soon after, I planned to deliver at home. I must admit that I was entirely skeptical—it sounded like a bit of a fad to me, and my feeling was that if womankind had been managing to have babies perfectly well for millennia, without a hundred and fifty bucks' worth of inflatable rubber involved, then I could do the same.

Added to my new way of thinking about birth was the advice, which I heard consistently, "If you like having a bath for period pain, then you will like water birth." I didn't really get period pain, but on the rare occasions I did, I was more of a hot water bottle under the duvet kind of girl. I decided against a pool. Besides, it would barely fit in our tiny living room, and I feared, even if it did, my birthing bottom might be rather too near the letter box for my liking.

In the end, the thought and planning I put into my first home birth was largely wasted, as I fell into the infamous induction trap. I was only a few days overdue, but the pressure I felt from those around me was so intense that I think it's unlikely I could ever have gone into labor naturally.

Eventually, tearful, uncomfortable, and desperate to do the right thing, I agreed to be induced in hospital, and my beautiful daughter Bess was born eighteen days after her estimated due date.

My labor was intense, but I chose not to have pain relief, and instead chanted a lot and spent some time in the large hospital bath. Everything seemed to be going well until, toward the end, it was decided that things were taking too much time. A man in a suit was called, and after an examination that I found incredibly traumatic, he declared she was "OP", or "back to back." My labor ended with feet in stirrups, an episiotomy, and a brief forceps delivery. Looking at the notes now, it is clear that the birth was pretty imminent when this happened, and with the beauty of hindsight, I do rather wish that those in charge of my care had put their efforts into helping me into new positions and feeding me a bit of banana, rather than resorting to what always seems to me a rather medieval solution to the "problem."

In spite of the trauma, I bonded and breastfed well with my daughter, although I think I was more than usually anxious in my first few months of motherhood, due in part to my feeling shell-shocked from the somewhat rough and forced nature of her beginning. But as time went by, I did begin to dwell a little less on what had happened, and it wasn't until I became pregnant again two years later, that my thoughts turned back to birth. Weirdly, although I was a mother already, there were two things I felt I had never done: gone into labor and pushed a baby out. So, I began to worry—was I actually capable of doing either of these things?

I decided to rethink water birth. By this time, quite a few friends had given birth in pools and they all raved about it. Added to this, we had moved to a larger house where fitting a birthing pool would be more practically possible, so I planned a home water birth with National Health Service (NHS) midwives. However, quite a long way into my pregnancy, my local midwifery system changed from community midwifery to a bank system, and I discovered that I might be attended by a midwife with no experience of home or water birth.

Since I had such doubts in my own capabilities, I wanted to be sure that my midwife, at least, knew what she was doing. We took the decision to hire an independent midwife, which turned out to be one of the best choices we ever made. The one-on-one care they offered meant they had time to help me process my first daughter's birth and prepare myself for a different experience. Their attitude toward birth was filled with confidence, and they filled me with confidence, too. They also didn't bat an eye when I went nearly two weeks past my due date.

However, that time of waiting was difficult. I felt huge, cumbersome, and, worst of all, riddled with doubt. I feared that there was something wrong with me, a switch missing that meant I would never go into labor spontaneously. As each day passed, I became more and more despondent. In spite of this, I did manage to avoid all of the natural induction methods that I had become caught up in last time. Instead, I focused on what I felt may be psychological blocks that were holding me back. I developed a mantra, "I am ready to let go," which seemed a good antidote to the anxious control freak aspect of my personality. I bounced on my birth ball, letting the baby's head knock on the door of my cervix, and repeated it over and over.

In the early hours of the morning on May 27th, I was woken by some very strong sensations. I had been asleep with my daughter, Bess, so I crept away to my partner George and woke him up. Could something be happening? We went downstairs together in the dark and chatted and waited for more and wondered what to do. The tightening feelings were intermittent, and eventually we put in a quick call to our midwife, Chrissy, who advised we go back to bed.

The next morning, there still seemed to be some activity, but it was patchy. Some sensations felt powerful, others like Braxton Hicks, and there was no real pattern. As we had an immersion tank hot water system, we decided to start filling the pool, just in case, as we had already had a trial run that had taken several hours.

By late morning there was still not much happening, and, of course, I remained full of doubt in my body and convinced it would all just fizzle out as I had experienced with my first pregnancy. I felt extremely hungry and had a huge, sudden craving for a fry up that absolutely had to include sausages. My lovely partner obeyed with a trip to the butcher. After my desire for "pig and egg" had been sated, I took myself off to bed for a nap.

When I woke, I felt different. Somehow, I just knew this was it. I went to the bathroom and tied my hair back. I can remember thinking (rather vainly) that I had better make an effort to make it look nice as I would be having my picture taken later holding my baby!

While I had been asleep, George had tidied up the house and put a vase of fresh lilac on the kitchen table, which I found very touching. He also started making vegetable soup—it all sounds idyllic, right? As he finely diced zucchini, I found myself having a really serious, I-mean-business contraction, kneeling on the floor of the living room, leaning on an armchair, with the two-year-old climbing on my back, and the dog, who never likes to be left out, placing a slobbery ball in front of my face.

I'm afraid I shattered the moment by yelling at the top of my lungs, "Stop making f*cking soup and get rid of this f*ucking dog!"

Suddenly, we both realized that something really was happening. The dog was banished to our neighbors. George's sister, Caroline, came to take care of Bess. The midwives were called. I lit some candles and put on some music. By myself in the living room, this felt like a good moment. I was actually in labor! I didn't have a missing switch, after all! And all this time the pool was sitting ready, kept warm by a cover, but I didn't want to get in until the midwives arrived. They had a long distance to come, over an hour's drive, and I was worried that the pool would speed up my labor and result in the midwives missing the birth! Whether or not this would have been the case, we will never know, but I was happy to err on the side of caution as I desperately wanted their presence.

Time passed, and the midwives did not arrive. My labor intensified. The midwives rang to say they were stuck in traffic. I kept trying to chant, as I had in my first labor, but somehow it just didn't work. It felt like wasted energy. Just before 6:00 p.m., I was on the sofa, struggling to find comfort and feeling really panicked by the absence of midwives. George was with me, and I started to cry. Where were they? And then, suddenly, they both came through the back door, their arms outstretched in reassurance and comfort. They both put their hands on me, they were warm and motherly, and I suddenly felt that everything would be alright.

After briefly checking me and the baby, they suggested I get in the pool. That was by far one of the most wonderful moments of my life. I felt as if the pain and anxiety was simply washed away by the water. In that moment, I realized water birth is not just a fad, and it's not really about pain relief, like having a bath when you've got your period. It's far deeper than that—it's a sanctuary, a place of safety, a watery nest where no one can reach you and where power is rightfully restored.

It's funny how my time in the pool was only an hour and three quarters, yet it's really my only true memory of labor. For those couple of hours, I felt as if all my perceptions were heightened, like moving from black and white to technicolor. Suddenly, I was able to gracefully flip my enormously pregnant body into whatever position felt best. My midwife, Chrissy, knelt by the pool and helped me through each contraction, guiding me in a low, gentle tone, which was just what I needed. I really was in my element.

The room seemed to be full of lightness and love. At one point, I asked Chrissy if she had dropped a torch in the pool, as it seemed suddenly illuminated in an otherwise fairly dark room. She hadn't, but a chink of light from the Spring evening sunshine had come through the curtains, striking the pool at just the right angle and making it glow an ethereal blue. We all marveled at this for some time, and even took photos. It felt like a nod of approval from Mother Nature herself.

Shortly after that my daughter returned from a walk with her Aunty. She had brought me a bunch of hedgerow flowers: cow parsley, buttercups, and red campion. I had been worried about what to do with her during a home birth, but it couldn't have been lovelier than to have her around, dipping in and out of the birth room and reminding me of what I was working toward. I felt huge waves of love for her, for my partner, and for everyone present!

Emotions ran high and deep. In the midst of all the love, I was working through my fears and trauma from my previous birth. I began to feel that the pushing stage was imminent, and this frightened me. I was scared I couldn't do it, and scared that I could! What would it feel like? It seemed an impossible feat. I really cried and the midwives and George gave me much needed reassurance.

My waters did not break until right near the end, in the pool. I also had a wee once or twice in the water. I highly recommend this to all water birthers – it feels a bit odd, but it is well diluted by the pool and it certainly beats what must be an agonizing trip to the loo. To give birth we really need to let go of concerns about what others think of us or what we should or shouldn't do. Weeing in the pool was quite liberating in this respect for me.

And then the pushing stage began: the ultimate in letting go. I was not a quiet birther who breathed her baby down into the world in tranquility. I roared. I gripped hard onto George's arms, he gripped mine, I knelt and I pulled back on his arms with all my might while I roared. I felt extremely powerful and completely determined.

If I could have talked, I might have shouted, "You are not going to get me this time, you f*ckers!"

I felt I was taking on the demons of my first birth trauma in that moment; reclaiming the strength they had briefly taken from me.

Chrissy asked me if I wanted to catch the baby. To me this seemed like a ridiculous suggestion!

"No! I'm . . . too . . . busy," I remember saying, so she gently passed her up to me through the water.

We looked to see what we had—a girl.

I held her, repeating incredulously, "I did it! I did it!"

I couldn't believe that it was over and that I had done it all myself. I felt elated.

I was aware that the midwives were repeating to me to rub my baby, and to talk to her, as if they were perhaps a little concerned, but I knew that she was fine. She soon began to make more visible signs of breathing, and suddenly my other daughter was in the room, and everyone was marveling in excitement at the new person present. George ripped off his clothes and jumped in the water to be closer to us, and Bess was helped out of her pajamas so she could do the same. It was an incredible moment between the four of us: a woman empowered and a family made new, in the very healing waters.

Truman's Birth Story

○ ○ ○ ○ ○ ○ ○ ○ ○ ○ ○ ○ ○ ○ ○ ○ ○ (○

"In my journal where I wrote out pieces of this story in the days following the birth, I tearfully describe how safe, loved, and supported I felt by my birth team. But I also describe fear: fear of pain, of the power of the pushy contractions, of something being wrong with the baby, of needing to transfer to the hospital. But I never let that fear become my focus during labor. I would note its presence, and then consciously let it go."
—Tracy, marriage and family therapist
Los Gatos, California

Truman's birth story begins with waiting. He was born just two days' shy of forty-two weeks, which, in California, is the cut-off date for legally having a midwife-attended home birth. Contractions started early on Friday morning. Then they stopped. They started again on Saturday and stopped again. By Sunday night I was in tears, wondering if this baby would ever arrive and if we would be able to have the home birth we had planned for. My dear husband, Andrew, helped lighten the mood and celebrate baby's impending arrival by packing a champagne picnic, our glow-in-the-dark bocce balls, and walking me down the lane behind our house for an impromptu evening celebration. I went to bed that night lighthearted (and light headed), trusting that all would be well.

On Monday, Andrew drove us from our secluded, rural home in the redwood forest into town for chiropractor and acupuncture appointments, both intended to start labor. By the time we headed home that afternoon, contractions were coming regularly and getting stronger by the minute. I wonder if we're one of the few home birth stories to begin with laboring mothers breathing through contractions in the car on the drive home, rather than a hospital birth where you're managing contractions on the way to the hospital!

Our midwife suggested that I eat some food, take a hot shower, and get some rest. I tried to eat, but food was totally unappealing to me. In the shower, I thought about the cervix, and its relationship to the throat. I sang the Indigo Girls song "Galileo" in the shower and thought about the song's messages of reincarnation and karma, and wondered about this little being on his way and the birth journey ahead. I remember my voice sounding sure and strong.

The shower didn't slow contractions or allow any rest. Instead, contractions became more intense and more frequent. I tried to get comfortable in bed and relax, but it wasn't too much later that I had my husband call our doula to have her head over. This part of the night is a blur, but I do know that right as our doula walked in the door, I was on the toilet and in the midst of a huge contraction. I felt something slip from between my legs. I was just fast enough to reach with my fingers and feel the sensation of a water balloon passing below me. My water had just broken.

Our doula helped me get going with the tens-unit while my husband got the birth tub ready. I started to find my rhythm through contractions, breathing and moaning, as our doula supported my lower back and swayed with me. I remember how reassuring her touch was for me at that moment. There were no doubts that I would be supported on the journey ahead.

I was relieved when the tub was filled and ready for me. We walked upstairs together, I stripped off my clothes, and submerged myself in the warm water. I found a comfortable position on my knees, leaning forward on the edge of the tub. Between contractions I would lay my head down on the side of the tub, close my eyes, and rest. As each new surge came upon me, I would begin to exhale deeply, signaling to Andrew and our doula that another contraction was on its way.

While in the birth tub, with candles lit, the room softly glowing, and my "labor-land" play list coming through the speakers, I lost all sense of time. With total darkness outside, I drifted between surges. I rested my head on the side of the tub, took sips of water, listened to encouraging words, felt firm touches, all while again and again riding waves of contractions. I found a rhythm with my breath, through moaning and growling, and our doula's encouragement to "bring it dowwwn" when my voice would reach for a higher pitch, and to "ooopen, open to your baby."

Suddenly, the urge to push came out of nowhere. But with a strong contraction, my body was instinctively bearing down. Our doula and Andy each made calls to our midwife to urge her to come. I remember our midwife as she arrived, leaning down next to me and saying quietly in my ear, "I'm here, Sweetie."

I had very little awareness of our midwives, but I knew they were there setting up for the birth and monitoring our baby's heart tones. As each movement would bring on another strong contraction, I would reluctantly move my leg or shift my body to allow our midwife to listen. In my journal, where I wrote out pieces of this story in the days following the birth, I tearfully describe how safe, loved, and supported I felt by my birth team. But I also describe fear: fear of pain, of the power of the pushy contractions, of something being wrong with the baby, of needing to transfer to the hospital. But I never let that fear become my focus during labor. I would note its presence, and then consciously let it go.

Back and forth between the birth tub and the bathroom, the contractions rocked my body along the way. I stood and held my husband's shoulders while swaying through each surge. I let myself get lost in the labor land trance, no self-consciousness, no shame, just going for the ride. My exhale blew orange poppy blossoms across a green field, like fogging up a mirror. Sacred symbols of the feminine, my female ancestors, and women everywhere were lending me strength as the night wore on.

No one ever checked my dilation. I was never told to push. My body took over with animal instinct, knowing exactly what to do. As the contractions became more intense and the pushing more regular, our doula sat in front of me on the floor and reached her hands into mine at each contraction. I would breath and squeeze her hands as I rode the incredible waves crashing over my body. Her hands were such a gift. They kept me grounded, gave me focus, and anchored me in the fierce storm.

Eventually our midwife suggested that I get up and go to the bathroom to pee. Even though I was reluctant to move (movement brought on painful surges), I followed her advice. The team dried me off and led me to the bathroom. Instead of our doula's support in the bathroom, this time Andy stayed with me. He stood in front of me as I sat on the toilet and rested my head on his hips. And for the first time in the night, I looked up at him and said, "This is so hard!"

He held his gaze on mine and said, "I know, baby. And you're doing such a great job."

Suddenly a huge contraction wracked my body. I gripped Andy's hips and moaned as an intense sensation of opening took over. I thought to myself, *if this isn't the ring of fire, I don't know what is!* I reached down between my legs and felt the baby's head emerging.

I shouted, "The baby's head is coming out!"

And suddenly, everyone was in our little bathroom. Our midwife placed the birth stool in front of the toilet and helped me scoot forward onto it.

She looked over at Andy and said, "Okay, are you ready to catch your baby?"

My next contraction was less pronounced, and I breathed through it to gently push again. Truman's head had emerged most of the way. I reached down again to feel his head. I looked over at Andy with surprise and delight. Wow! This is the moment we had been waiting for! With just two or three more pushes our baby was born. I pulled him to my chest and listened to his first cries. Incredible!

Not too long after, our midwife looked up at me and said, "Tracy, I need you to stop bleeding now."

I took my focus from the baby in my arms and brought it inside of myself. I firmed up the outward pushing energy of my abdomen and clamped down internally. Once our midwife was satisfied that I was okay to move, the whole gang helped me up and walked me over to the couch, Truman still attached to the umbilical cord and the placenta still inside me.

On the couch, I held Tru to my chest while our midwife inspected my body. After a period of time, she gave me a piece of gauze to grip the umbilical cord and with a gentle tug and a whoosh, my placenta was delivered.

The rest of the night was captured more by photographs than by my journal notes. I think we all rested on the couch together for at least an hour before Andy cut the umbilical cord. After that, our birth team helped me into the shower while Andy held Truman. Filled with adrenaline and fatigue, I was so shaky that I needed help to stand and wash in the shower, and I needed their help every step of the way to bed.

At this point, the sky was starting to turn from pitch black to light gray, the outlines of treetops becoming visible against the sky. We journeyed through the night together and made it to morning. Tears streamed down my face as our doula embraced me and told me how strong I was. My heart burst with love as I looked at Andrew, knowing we had experienced this incredible event together. Truman lay quietly on the bed between us; his dark eyes wide open to the new world surrounding him.

A Gentle Birth

○ ○ ○ ○ ○ ○ ○ ○ ● ○ ○ ○ ○ ○ ○ ● ○

"Even now, typing up Odhran's birth story, I am in tears remembering my powerful birth experience. I feel blessed and honored to have been able to tap into and experience this part of myself. I know it probably sounds corny, but it feels like I accessed a connection to a powerful goddess in me."

—Mary, doula and GentleBirth instructor
Midleton, Co. Cork, Ireland

My estimated due date was the 29th of July, nine days later than the twelve-week hospital scan. However, I had been charting my own cycle, and I was completely confident that my due date was more accurate. As a result, I had politely, but firmly, argued with the hospital that I would not accept the scan date as my due date. I really didn't want to have the pressure of induction that I had faced with my first birth, Sadbh's, a few years back; that event was still very much in my mind. I was glad I advocated for my more accurate due date as the 20th of July came and went, as did my own estimated due date.

For this pregnancy, I was not as fearful as with my first. In general, my panic attacks had improved, and they were not as debilitating as when I was pregnant with Sadbh. I had also experienced a really positive birth experience, and I also knew a lot more about how Gentle Birth worked, as I was now teaching monthly workshops in Cork. There was still some fear, though. The fact that I was teaching the workshops was a stress as I felt under pressure to have a positive birth experience. I couldn't help but think that perhaps the first-time 'round I was just lucky and this time I would see how birth really was: painful and excruciating. (I mean that's what most people had told me it was going to be like, so maybe they were right!) It is amazing how strong fear can be and how much the brain can hold onto fear. I went back to listening to my Gentle Birth tracks and, like the last time, I instantly felt at peace and more positive. For the residual fear, I listened to the "Fear Release" track over and over. I also brought my husband, David, through the Gentle Birth workshop so he could learn and understand the helpful tools tailored for expectant dads. Although this was an education for David, it also helped me feel confident that he would understand where I was during the birth and knew how to support me.

On Saturday, the 31st of July, I did my usual Saturday routine: I went down to the local market to shop for food for the week, bumping into lots of friends on the way for a chat. All were surprised I was still "hanging in there." (I was enormous during this pregnancy!) I felt perhaps labor was starting; I had been getting what felt like very mild tightening in my abdomen all morning. However, I wasn't sure, as they were so mild I felt they could have been warm-up surges (Braxton Hicks). After shopping and lunch, I went for an acupuncture appointment and explained to my acupuncturist, the amazing Pierce Hennessy in Midleton who had been treating me for the entire pregnancy, that I could be in labor. I had a lovely treatment and listened to my Gentle Birth CD while on the table. The treatment took about forty minutes, and I took note that I had three surges while there. They were still extremely mild. They still just felt like tightening sensations, but they did seem to be getting slightly stronger. After acupuncture, I went downtown to do a few more bits and pieces before making my way home.

I went up to rest in bed for a while and debated whether to call my friend, Tracey, who was on my support team for the birth. She lives in Tipperary, about a two hours' drive away, and was due to come down the next day for a visit. Eventually, my gut told me to phone her, which I did. I explained my hesitation, but she said she would leave right away. I then went back up to bed and watched some TV. During a trip to the toilet I had what seemed like a minuscule show. I tried to temper my excitement.

Around 6:00 p.m., my four-year-old daughter, Sadbh, and husband, David, came home from a birthday party. I greeted Sadbh with a huge pillow fight upstairs. I was still having surges, and they seemed to be getting stronger as I found myself having to stop playing for a second in order to breathe through each surge. Then, around 7:00 p.m., Tracey and my other friend, Gwen (who was staying locally) arrived. These two friends along with my Mam and David were my birth team. We all sat down to a lovely dinner cooked by David and washed it down with some Prosecco (but not too much!). It was a great evening with rounds of joking and laughing, ending in us all dancing around the kitchen to my daughter's favorite song, "All the Single Ladies."

By this stage, the surges were definitely getting stronger. I had to stop eating and talking to breathe through each one. I still wasn't sure if I was in labor, however, as each surge was manageable. Gwen suggested I call Mary Cronin (my midwife) just to let her know I was having surges and how close they were (about every fifteen minutes). Then we all went into the sitting room to watch a Tom and Jerry DVD with Sadbh. After about a half an hour of the DVD, I had to leave the room. The surges were intensifying and Tom and Jerry was a bit too active for me! I had continued to use deep breathing during each surge and was feeling great. Myself, Gwen, Tracey, and David went upstairs and set up the laptop to watch Glee—I had been saving episodes to watch during labor. After about twenty minutes my waters released (this was about 10:40 p.m.). I phoned the midwife who said she was on her way. After my waters went, the surges intensified. I still felt in control and the contractions were manageable. I knew I had picked the perfect birth team as David, Tracey, and Gwen were making me laugh so much that the intensity of each surge would simply dissipate with the laughter.

After a while the surges became very powerful so I got up on my birth ball and rolled. My doulas rubbed my back in between each contraction with a lovely aromatherapy mix, which felt and smelled great, and helped me relax. Gwen rubbed me down with a cool cloth, as I was feeling extremely hot (needless to say I had stopped watching Glee at this stage). After a while I began to feel like I needed to vomit, and asked for a bucket. Thankfully this sensation passed quickly without a need for the bucket. All the while I was listening to my Gentle Birth CD. It is hard to accurately put into words how I really felt. I have heard and read stories from women who say they enter this powerful zone where their body is doing all the work. I suppose it is like what it says in the Gentle Birth workshop: turn your thinking brain off.

Ina May Gaskin says about birth, "Let your monkey do it."

Well, this is how it felt: my thinking brain was in me somewhere, but it was hard to access. Putting a sentence together was terribly challenging. At one point, I wanted a hair band, but I found it impossible to formulate the request. I had managed to access this powerful, primal part of myself, and it felt amazing. All of my body was busy birthing my baby, and I felt full of power, so much a woman, so connected to that primitive part of me that just knew how to birth this baby. I didn't have to do anything; my body was working effectively.

The surges were taking over completely, like waves coursing through my body, ebbing and flowing from my head to my toes. They were intense and powerful, but not painful.

I have no idea how frequently the contractions were coming on or the breaks between them. I did manage to ask to get the pool filled as I wanted to float in water. I thought the water would be a chance to rest my legs, which were suffering from edema. I asked Tracey and Gwen to fill it, as I wanted David upstairs with me. At 11:40 p.m., the midwife arrived and examined me. She put the lights on, but I couldn't bear them. They were promptly turned off. I found out later I was nine centimeters at this stage. I didn't ask that night as I didn't want to know and didn't even think to ask.

I do remember at times thinking that the surges were so strong I would not be able to handle the next one. However, the other part of my brain would kick in and override the doubt and go with what was happening to my body. All the time I had the Gentle Birth CD on, and this helped immensely, as I associated it with relaxation and calmness. The affirmations were also great.

At some point my daughter came into the room to see me. David explained to her that I was having the baby and that although I was being very vocal, I wasn't in pain.

"I know," Sadbh replied.

She was not a bit phased by me in labor. She sat down on the bed beside David and ten minutes later, she was asleep.

David was a great help as well; reminding me to breathe and telling me how amazing I was. His affirmations were reassuring, reminding me that I could birth our baby. A short time after the midwife arrived, we transferred downstairs. I was still hoping to use the pool. I had no idea how dilated I was, but the surges felt different. Each contraction felt more like I was bearing down so I presume I was in the second stage of labor. I don't remember walking downstairs. The sitting room was dark, but the pool was nowhere near ready. I knelt on the couch for a while with David supporting me. Then I went and sat on the birth stool I had borrowed from a friend. Thank goodness for it, as it helped so much with my swollen legs, and had a lovely cushion. I leaned into David, who was on a chair. I didn't realize it, but at this stage the baby's head was at my perineum, and I was trying to push him out. Forty minutes later (around 1:15 am), we were still in the same boat: the baby's head at my perineum, but he couldn't get past it. My perineum just wouldn't stretch to let him out. Toward the end of this period I did start to feel pain. He was pressing against my bladder, and I felt like I needed to pee but couldn't. I was panicking a bit, because in my first labor I had been in second stage labor for over twelve hours at home before needing to be transferred to hospital. Our midwife encouraged me to reach down and feel our baby's head. This seemed to be a replay of what had happened with Sadbh's birth, and I didn't want to have the same experience again. I don't think I realized how different this birth was, as Odhran was just about ready to be born. Unlike my previous birth, the surges were powerful, but he just could not get past my perineum.

I asked the birth team to go into the kitchen. Perhaps everyone watching was slowing me down. To no avail. The midwife had me change position to widen my legs. Again, no joy. She tried to help me stretch and give the baby some more room to pass with her fingers. No luck. Eventually, she suggested an episiotomy. After consulting with the other midwife, Ellmarie, they all agreed an episiotomy was the best option, and so I agreed to it. I was hesitant since I had an episiotomy last time as well, and I was really hoping to avoid another. However, our midwifes could not think of anything else to do at this stage, so I agreed to it and she gave me a small cut first. No baby. She then widened the cut. It took another two or three surges and the baby's head finally came out. It felt amazing! Now I reached down and felt my baby's head. With the next surge, our baby's body came out; it was so long, and it felt so warm. I took my little boy in my arms and felt exhilarated. Here I was holding my new son in my arms: I felt like a warrior. I was on a high. I hobbled over to the couch (the cord was still attached) and laid down holding our baby in my arms. He was so warm and wet and gorgeous. The rest is a blur. Mary let the cord pulsate for a few minutes, then cut it as she had to get cord blood (I am Rhesus Negative). David cut the cord. Then we waited for the placenta to birth.

Mary sewed me up as we opened a bottle of champagne to celebrate. The birth team got busy cleaning up the house and cleaning me up, as well. We were all on a high. Although Odhran was born at 1:31 a.m., we didn't go to bed until 5:30 a.m.; I was high on hormones and excitement after such an amazing birth. Even now, typing up Odhran's birth story, I am in tears remembering my powerful birth experience. I feel blessed and honored to have been able to tap into and experience this part of myself. I know it probably sounds corny, but it feels like I accessed a connection to a powerful goddess in me.

We named our son Odhran, and he weighed nine pounds and fifteen ounces. He started breastfeeding soon after. One of the first things I said to David after he was born (before the cord was even cut) was, "Oh, I need to do that again! Can we have a third one?" For such a short birth, this certainly is a long birth story, but I wanted to remember it all and capture every detail in words. Like my first labor, I found the Gentle Birth program incredibly helpful. During my pregnancy, the CDs helped to allay any fears I had. It also gave me the chance to take some time for myself every day; with a four-year-old and working outside the home part-time, it was a challenge to find the time, but it was so worth it. When my labor started, I felt excitement rather than fear. This allowed me to trust my body to birth my baby.

Chapter 8

Let's Hear It for the Dads

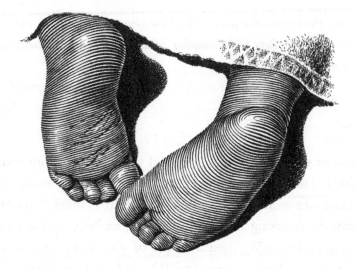

Oscar and Karolina:
From IVF to Home Birth

○ ○ ○ ○ ○ ○ ○ ○ ● ● ● ○ ● ○ ○ ● ● ○

"The moral of this story is that you can do all the planning in the world, but in the end, you need to be flexible, adapt to the situation, make sure that mom is comfortable, and do whatever she says at all costs."

—Oscar, network analyst
Maryland

After a year of trying to conceive a child, I was diagnosed with male infertility in 2008. This killed our chances at having our own biological child, but it did not take away the desire that we had. After many years of trying to go down the fostering and adoption route, we came across a program for adopting embryos. We tried a couple of different programs and did several transfers with no success. In 2012, we found a new program, and after much discernment, made the choice to go with them and transfer two embryos in early 2013, with one successfully implanting. My wife, Karolina was, and still is, a huge advocate for empowering women. We talked and decided that a home birth would be perfect for her. I agreed since I myself was born at home in El Salvador. We found a great midwife office that did both home births as well as midwifery care at a birth center. We figured that we had options and that was good.

As we got closer to the due date, we started taking birthing classes (Hypnobabies), breastfeeding classes, and tours of hospitals. We started creating our very detailed birth plans and got the birth room ready. (It's always a great time arguing with a pregnant woman about what she will need or want during the birth.) We decided to go with the Hypnobabies birth training and a birth pool for Karolina to relax in. We made plans with our vet to drop off our two beagles no matter the time of day. We made a list of snacks to have on hand. Most importantly, we discussed when we would start taking visitors after baby was born, how long they could stay, and who would kick them out. I was assigned the bad guy role, which was fine with me.

The morning of November 25th, Karolina woke up with cramps, but nothing too crazy. We agreed that it was probably a good time to get the pool set up, go grocery shopping, and get ready in case the baby decided to come soon. Around noon, in our endless wisdom, we decided that I should go into the office, submit my time sheets, and set my out-of-office message on my email. Did I mention that my round-trip work commute was three hours? Or that it was right before Thanksgiving? I made it to the office, submitted my paperwork, said Merry Christmas and Happy New Year to everyone since I was not planning on coming back for a while. Yes, I know, a whole month. Why? Because I wanted to be with my wife and child for as long as I could, and I was blessed with having the ability to do so.

Around 4:00 p.m. I left the office and started my trek home. As usual, traffic was bumper to bumper from Baltimore to Washington, DC. Around 5:00 p.m. I was entering the DC beltway when Karolina called to inform me that her water had broken. @*$(*&#$(, I say. At this point I was still a good hour away in that traffic. My heart started to pound faster. I listened to the traffic report, trying to find alternate routes, but everything was backed up. Alas, I finally got home. Remember that birth tub that we set up in the morning? Well, we had not filled it yet. After all, the baby was not supposed to be coming this fast. I got the hose and attached it to the bathroom sink. All good to go, I thought to myself. After several minutes, I went to check the temperature of the water, and it was cold. What the hell? Oh, yes, we are thrifty/green people so we had lowered the water heater temperature and never turned it back up for this event.

It was 8:00 p.m. the birth team was now on site, and I told them about the tub situation. They suggested that I boil water on the stove and carry it upstairs to the pool room. So, in between water runs, I was trying to keep Karolina calm and focused during her contractions. Needless to say, I was failing on all fronts. I am guessing that I looked lost in all of this, so our midwife, Jennifer, suggested abandoning the birth pool altogether. My wife was not happy about this, but I took the hit and disconnected the hose so that people would not trip and fall down the stairs. I was finally able to focus on what Karolina needed.

It was now around 10:00 p.m. and the baby was coming. Karolina had not left the bathroom, as that was where she felt most comfortable. During one of the baby checks we could see that our baby was starting to crown. Wow, such an amazing and scary sight! Karolina decided that she wanted to be leaning over her birthing ball, so we moved to the bedroom. It did not take long before the baby's head was coming, followed by the rest of the body. It was so fast that our baby slipped through Jennifer's hands and landed on the bed. As soon as we could get Karolina to lay down, we put our baby on her belly. Jennifer informed us that the cord had stopped pulsating and that we should cut it. I got the pleasure of cutting it and wrapping our baby up. There was a lot of bleeding. Suddenly my wife started to go into shock so I took our baby and went to the pool room to allow Jennifer to take care of her. After what seemed like forever, she was finally stable and I came back into the room with our baby. We still did not know the sex of our baby! At this point, I looked for the first time.

I turned to my wife and said, "Honey, meet your daughter, Natalia Maya."

We both cried, hugged, and kissed our beautiful, still covered in vernix daughter.

The moral of this story is that you can do all the planning in the world, but in the end, you need to be flexible, adapt to the situation, make sure that mom is comfortable, and do whatever she says at all costs. As eventful as this birth was, I would do it all over again (and actually, we did, just a few weeks ago!).

Rockstar Dad

o o o o o o O o o o o o o o o o (o

"She was magnificent in the glory of child birth, and I got to witness it."
—Brendan, Rockstar Dad
Melbourne, Australia

As a man, I have to say, childbirth is pretty daunting. In fact, deep down I harbor the viewpoint of the men-of-old that childbirth "is a woman's business." My parents had five children, and my father attended only one birth (mine) and he "attended" it from the hospital waiting room. He never even made it inside the hospital for the other four births as he was too busy holding down a job and looking after the kids, and, let's face it; what use was he gonna be? My mother always told me that his parting words as he dropped her at the hospital were, "call me when it's time to come and pick you up." Hmmm . . . the good ol' days!

I have four beautiful children today; two from my first marriage, ages eighteen and sixteen, and two from my second marriage, ages two and a half and one and a half. I have attended all their births, and when I say attended, I mean really attended, and I have had vastly different birth experiences; some harrowing, and some extremely beautiful.

I did not try to influence how my partners wanted to birth our children (hospital vs. home, drugs vs. none, etc.). I basically left it up to them to decide what worked for them, and then I went with the flow, and I still stand by that approach. After all, they were the ones giving birth, they had the right to make the decision on how they wanted to do it.

My first child was a breech baby and was delivered by Cesarean. At the time, I thought, *Great!* as I was totally petrified of spending long hours in a hospital room with my wife in a lot of pain. A Cesarean seemed the easy way out (so to speak). As a modern-day father, I had attended all the prenatal classes, learned the breathing techniques, knew how to give a massage, etc., but deep down I knew when push came to shove I was going to be totally useless in the labor ward. I cannot say I really embraced those classes; I did not really understand what was going on except that we were having a baby, and in the pecking order of doctor, nurse, hospital janitor . . . I was clearly a distant last in influencing the successful birth of my child.

I was definitely not prepared. When the Cesarean started, all I knew was they were about to take a knife to my wife's tummy, open it up, and pull out our child. Here's me, sh*t-scared, and it's my poor wife who's having the actual operation. Jeez, how was she feeling? You know, I am not sure I really asked her. I probably did not want to know. Someone had to be brave, and it was certainly not me. Incessant talking was what I had to do during the operation. My wife was being cut open, and to take her mind from the sensation of tugging (which can induce panic), I was told I had to take her mind off the operation, so I talked like there was no tomorrow. What we gonna call the baby? Start reciting all those names we'd been thinking of. How should we spell Natasha? Maybe with an e, an i, or an o, and so forth. (Please note: any disagreement on baby names dissipates in a millisecond in that operating room. Your wife will always win.) The operation was over in minutes, and we had a daughter. I was handed the baby (for all my hard work), and my wife stayed in the operating theater for the next thirty minutes while they sewed her back up.

The feeling I had that day with our new baby was like nothing I had ever felt before. What Cesarean? What hospital? What sleep? We didn't care. My beautiful wife and I just wanted to party with our new daughter. Everything we/she had just gone through paled into insignificance once we had our newborn in our arms.

Round two, eighteen months later, and we were back in the same hospital. My wife was bravely opting for a vaginal birth this time, with the help of whatever drugs were needed. Small contractions had started three days prior. We had a busy toddler to look after, and my wife had gotten very little sleep, so she arrived at the hospital already exhausted. Again,

I felt totally unprepared and was back in the frame of mind of let's get this over and done with as soon as possible . . . please say Cesarean. Prior to the birth, I cannot really remember having any discussion about what we would do as a team to get this baby out. I guess I didn't feel like I was on the team. Don't get me wrong, I appear to be joking about my non-teaming approach, but reflecting back I think I was looking for someone to tell me what to do.

I should have been prepared, and I wasn't. It was a blood bath. Forceps, suction, cutting—I never ever wanted to see another child born in my whole life. What my wife went through that day was horrific. The number of drugs pumped into her to get her through left her shivering unconscious on the bed. The doctor told me to come and look at the business end as the baby came out, and I have to be honest, it was not pretty. Nothing could have prepared me for what happened that day to someone I love. The hospital seemed to be operating on a timed schedule, and they wanted that baby out by the end of the day—and get it out they did. But what a mess they made. It took my wife weeks to recover from stitching and hemorrhoids. Meanwhile, I had sat back and watched the whole thing and said nothing, because I felt like I knew nothing. My wife and I never really spoke about the trauma of the night, yet we should have. It needed discussing. What a woman will go through to have a baby is beyond my comprehension.

Fast forward fifteen years and I was back to where I never really wanted to be: preparing for a child birth. But it is amazing what time does to your memory and what a new love can talk you into. This birth was freaking me out a little bit, though, as it was going to be a home birth. My imagination ran away from me . . . *will we need new carpet and a lick of paint to remove the blood stains? Where do you have a Cesarean in a home birth? Will I ever be able to sit and watch the game on the couch if I witness a messy delivery on the lounge room floor?* Already I'm thinking we were going to have to move house.

We sat through two Sundays of a Calm Birth course (I would be calmer if they held it in the pub), but I already knew there was nothing calm about birth. I figured we would be sitting with a bunch of hippies smoking pot, discussing home birth, garden birth, minivan birth, but the class turned out to be made up of twelve other couples from various backgrounds. The main thing I noticed was that the soon-to-be mothers were all very calm and focused. Having a home birth or natural birth with no drugs was their focus, and they were ready for it. The men were less vocal. Some seemed to have embraced it fully, where others, i.e., me, maintained a healthy skepticism. Three things I came away with from the Calm Birth course were: it's pressure, not pain (who're you kidding, you're talking to a pro), you need a birth plan, and most importantly, when it's all getting hard, man, you have to step up, take control, and be involved. It's your wife, your child. Be a *man*.

The pressure of childbirth has since been described to me "like running a marathon." Instead of focusing on the pain, it's more about endurance, stamina, mental toughness, and self-belief. Birthing women have this in abundance, so much more than men. I've had the privilege of seeing the two loves of my life, my first and second wives, demonstrate this toughness well beyond any sporting star I have watched on TV. In fact, maybe that's the fear of birth for men—that it will show our inadequacies. I certainly showed mine in my first two births.

After Calm Birth, I certainly felt a little less apprehensive about the impending birth. I'm not a hippy-loving home birth dude; I still felt that I could happily skip the birth and come into the room with a bottle of champagne two minutes later, but I was not quite so scared anymore. Preparing for a home birth is a little different than just packing your hospital bag. My wife was very calm and had lists to cover it all. Music was selected, shower curtains to protect the furniture, blankets to birth upon, a blow-up pool big enough for the kids to swim in, even a pooper-scooper if required for the pool (don't ask). I feel like I'm totally winging it and will be likely drinking a beer and standing in the corner when the time comes.

It was 2:00 a.m., and it was *on*. My wife was laying on the couch having contractions for two hours while I got my beauty sleep. They were coming so close together that it was time to call in the midwives (that was me taking control). Now, these ladies were pretty cool, with a wicked sense of humor, and within thirty minutes all three of them were on the doorstep buzzing and excited (did they not realize it was 2:30 a.m.)?

So, I had three midwives, one pregnant wife, a six-year-old stepdaughter, and a sister-in-law all ready to watch/catch/participate (and again, I thought *why am I here?*). Quite frankly, testosterone does not deserve its place at a birth. I was Mr. cup-of-tea man, change-the-music man, forget-to-fill-the-pool man, make-a-piece-of-toast man, have-not-got-a-clue-where-anything-is man, will-we-really-need-the-pooper-scooper man. I am all of these things to the bevy of women in our house, and you know what? We were at home having a baby, and it was pretty cool. I felt pretty darn calm. All these women buzzing around making things happen and I felt in control, like the master of this domain.

Over the next four hours I got to be a part of a birth I had never experienced before—it was amazing, beyond amazing. Now the births of my first two children were certainly unreal, and the euphoria of holding your babe is second to none (although Ireland winning the World Cup might come close), but what was amazing about home birth was the process of the birth, the natural flow of the birth, and watching with the utmost admiration at how my wife was able to give birth in her own home, on her own terms (no stirrups for this gal). She was magnificent in the glory of childbirth, and I got to witness it. I cannot remember the mechanics of everything, but it just happened so naturally, without rushing or panic. Mr. pooper-scooper man wouldn't mind going through birth like that again.

And just twelve months later, I got my chance. Another home birth, this time, only two and a half hours in duration. The same midwives came through the door, gave us a kiss, asked for a cup of tea, and made themselves at home. My wife made labor look easy, but this time I was much more involved, much more of a key player. I read the situation, anticipating what she needed, holding her when it was required, giving her space when she needed it, putting the kettle on in between contractions; we were birthing this one together. Our beautiful babe was born in the shower just before midnight and an hour later I was snoring in bed. What's not to love?

So, take control, man. Your woman wants you to be confident, in control, supportive, and most of all to be there, in body and soul. I am not saying that home birth is always the go and I am also not professing to be Mr. natural-Calm Birth-dude, but what I experienced with my third and fourth births made me just a little bit more a man. If I had my chance again with my first two births, I would be more assertive and stop being a passenger. I would do what I needed to do. Yes, I would. Even if I was secretly thinking about running away to the pub and watching the game until it was all over.

Jeff from Colorado

○ ○ ○ ○ ○ ○ ○ ○ ● ● ○ ○ ○ ○ ○ ○ ● ●

"I don't know how to explain what I was feeling at that point, but it was a mixture of elation and relief, realizing the realness of a human being born, and the effort that goes into giving birth. And all of this, I didn't realize when my first son was born. It wasn't that he wasn't special to me, but I think it was that I was just disconnected from the experience even though I was right there."

—Jeff, science teacher
Colorado Springs, Colorado

My wife, Amye, and I were married in 2012. When we initially talked about having kids, we briefly mentioned having a home birth, but we didn't know anyone who had had a home birth or how it would go. We decided that since we didn't know much about home birth, we would just do the common thing and have a hospital birth. We did take a longer and more intense eight-week birth class that gave us a lot of great information; we felt prepared for the birth of our first child. After our first kid was born in a hospital, we reflected on the experience. It was good, except for a few hard things that we thought were completely normal. It wasn't until after we had a home birth that we looked back and realized how much better the first birth could have been if we had stayed home with a midwife.

We initially looked into having a home birth for financial reasons. Our insurance had changed, and we were shocked at how much we were going to pay out of pocket. My wife talked with our new insurance company, and they loved supporting families that do home births with a midwife. My wife did some initial research and interviewed a few midwives until we found one that we liked. We hired Kim when my wife was sixteen weeks pregnant, and we were surprised by the level of personal care that Amye and the baby received. It wasn't just a fifteen-minute visit. Kim was able to help with all aspects of pregnancy, including food, sleeping, rest, and exercise. Kim also took into account how Amye's previous birth affected her idea of what this birth would be like at home. We were scared of having another experience like we did in the hospital; the delivery and recovery were difficult. Kim assured us that she had a plan for us to be as prepared as possible for a more positive outcome for everyone.

Amye is a doula so she has some experience with how to be aware of the different signs of early labor. For our home birth, Amye went into labor at 3:00 a.m., and she instantly knew that this was "it." I called the midwife and Amye's doula, and everyone made it to our house in around fifteen minutes. Our midwife also brought along an assistant midwife and a midwife in training. They were familiar to us because they were at appointments, as well. They walked in calmly and quietly with a bunch of bags, which was reassuring. After about twenty minutes of knowing that Amye was in labor, our midwife thought it would be a good idea for Amye to labor in bed due to some of the signs she was seeing. Our bed was prepped and ready to go.

I was ready for the actual labor experience. This pregnancy was hard on Amye, and I was ready to meet our son, Jack. For each contraction, I was next to Amye on the bed. I was holding her hand, encouraging her, and assisting her in moving to new positions. I felt more connected to the birth process by being right there next to her instead of standing next to her in a hospital bed. While we had a doula, who would be there for back support as needed, I was my wife's main line of support. Contractions never got out of hand even during transition, and I think that was because we were in a very peaceful environment in our own home. We had our home cleaned the week before, and we kept it clean leading up to birth, and everything else was taken care of. There were no intrusive checks or people running around and coming in and out of the room. I knew these people that were in our room. I trusted them because I had known them for the last seven months, and knew what they were capable of. Our midwife knew exactly where the baby was and how the baby was doing, and encouraged Amye, as well.

There was a time where I had to go to the bathroom; it was the saddest thing to leave Amye for that short amount of time because I felt like I was needed more than anyone else in the room. It was such a different feeling from our first birth at the hospital, where I could have just held her hand and she wouldn't have known any different.

Then, the pushing stage came, and our midwife wanted to slow down the pushing a bit. At one point, we had talked about me catching Jack, and I was open to the idea. I knew for sure I wasn't trained in catching a baby, but I had held my previous son enough to know how to hold any baby. To tell the truth, I was so focused on supporting Amye that I had almost forgotten about catching Jack; Kim didn't forget. As I watched Jack move lower and lower, our midwife said for me to move over and take her spot. She slid over to my side and a bit behind me. If she would have asked me if I wanted to catch Jack, I would have hesitated and possibly even said, "Oh no, you can catch him," but Kim just slid over. I had to move into position. Can you imagine if I had asked the doctor who was in a full gown, face mask, and gloves during my first son's birth if they could move over so that I could catch the baby?

At this point, the sun had risen and it started to get light in the room. The birds were chirping. Even though Amye was about to deliver our child, there was never any fear in the room. It was peaceful. The pace and activity in the room never noticeably changed. Yes, the team prepped a few things here and there, but we never noticed. As I saw Jack crowning, it instantly became real.

I shouted to Amye, "I can see Jack! He is here! He is finally here! This is it!"

The culmination of many months of waiting for him to be here was nearly over and we would get to meet him in a few moments. This encouraged Amye greatly and made the pushing process easier. Once his head came far enough out, I touched his hard, slippery head for the first time and it instantly became even more real; so real and so much emotion all at once, that I completely lost it. I was balling my eyes out, and it was hard for me to encourage Amye through what was happening. I don't know how to explain what I was feeling at that point, but it was a mixture of elation and relief, realizing the realness of a human being born, and the effort that goes into giving birth. And all of this, I didn't realize when my first son, Hunter, was born. It wasn't that he wasn't special to me, but I think it was that I was just disconnected from the experience even though I was right there.

A couple pushes later, Jack was born. I caught him and brought him up to Amye to hold. At first I forgot that new born babies aren't as sturdy as eighteen month olds, and they are much more slippery. After about a half second, I realized this and got a proper hold of him and brought him to Amye. Together we got to laugh and cry and celebrate the birth of Jack. It was a special moment that I will never forget. I am so glad I didn't sit back and allow the professionals to do a job that I could do myself. I am not saying that I didn't need them, but they knew exactly what was the right thing to do at the time, and I am so glad they gave me the opportunity to catch our baby.

Jack was born at 6:00 a.m., and we had the rest of the day to relax and enjoy our new baby. Friends had picked up our dog at 3:30 in the morning, and another friend picked up our two-year-old who was just beginning to wake up at 6:00 a.m. Jack was with Amye for at least forty-five minutes just being held and nursing before the midwives did their newborn check. I couldn't believe there was so much less intervention than in a hospital. In the hospital, Amye did get to hold Hunter for a bit, but he was quickly taken away to be cleaned and bathed and checked, which took a bit of time. At home, we simply got to relish in the experience of birth and our new baby. Our midwives quietly exited the room and hung out in the living room to allow us to rest and call friends and family and spend time with Jack. It was amazing. It was quiet, we ate breakfast, and every forty-five minutes or so, Kim would check on us. We were prepared and had a tray of food for them to snack on, figuring they might be at our house for a bit.

After a couple hours, we had settled in and nothing else needed to be done but to relax in the quiet of our home with Jack.

We relaxed on the porch that evening and kept asking ourselves, "Did we really have a baby this morning?"

We couldn't get over the peacefulness of the experience of our own home. In the hospital, there were strangers coming into our room all the time. We were so ready to get home after two days with our first. For all the dads out there, the couch bed at the hospital is always six inches too short no matter how tall you are. Our friends brought Hunter back on the third day to join us as a family of four, and it was so much fun for him to meet his new brother.

I wish dads and expectant dads out there would take a little bit of time to understand the pros and cons of a home birth versus a hospital birth. Although we took the birth class with our first son, I really didn't know much about birth. Dads, you need to know that you are needed more than anyone else when your wife gives birth; you have a connection with her that no one else does. Talk with other dads who have had a home birth and/or a hospital birth. I never would have thought I would share my story about home birth in a book, but here I am. I want to share my story with every man who is going to be having kids.

I wish it was more acceptable to start conversations with friends, acquaintances, and coworkers by saying, "Hey, I am really glad we had a home birth, and I want to tell you everything about it so you might consider having a home birth as well!"

Don't settle for what society says is normal. Reach for what is best for you, your wife, and your family. I guarantee you will surprise yourself with what you are capable of experiencing as a family.

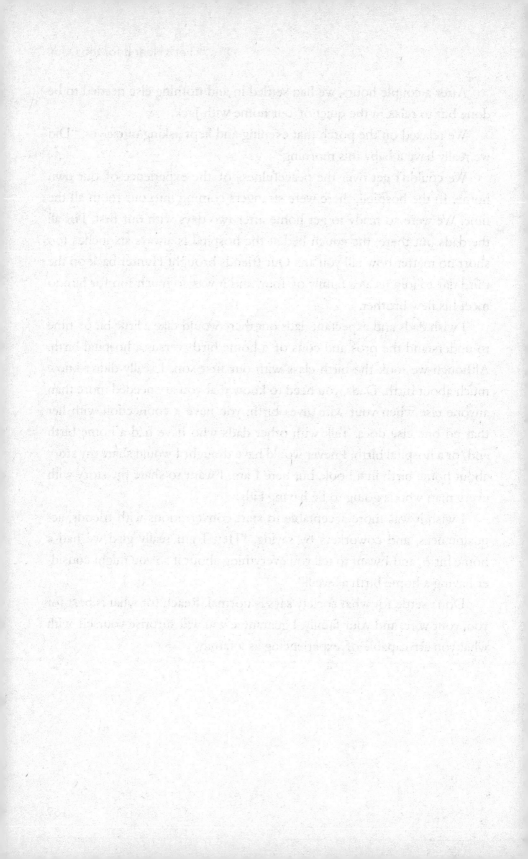

Chapter 9

Positive Hospital Transfers

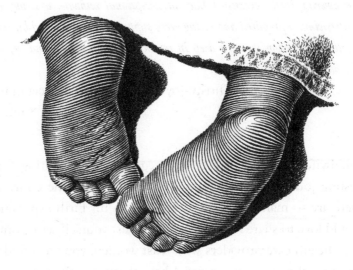

The Power of a
Supportive Birth Team

o ○ ○ O ○ ○ O ○ ○ • ○ ○ ○ ○ • ○ (○

"I had what would be called a difficult birth, but I didn't experience it as that. I had an empowering birth, because I had an exceptional midwife, a strong doula, a feminist obstetrician, a prepared and loving birth support team, a devoted husband, and a determination and knowing born deep in my being that my body and my baby are designed for birth."

—Christy-Joy Ras, registered nurse and midwife
Cape Town, South Africa

I am a midwife, which makes being pregnant and preparing for birth an interesting journey of comparison for myself and the entire experience. There are so many facets of wonder from my birth experience, but what I would love to share is this: when you trust yourself as a woman and you choose health care providers who trust women, you are gifted a birth experience that changes you forever. I have witnessed the power of birth many times, but the miracle and power of life was truly affirmed by my own experience giving birth. I planned a home birth, I negotiated for my home birth, and I was respected by the people around me. More important to me than where I birthed was where I labored. And I labored as I had envisioned: in a home environment with my chosen and prepared birth support team.

When I worked in Johannesburg as a midwife, I had the privilege of attending my first home birth with a woman named Sue King. Witnessing a baby born in a home environment changed everything for me, and I knew that one day, that was how I wanted to labor and birth. Sue was an incredible midwife and friend. She was a brave woman who listened to women's bodies and to her intuition to make informed decisions. She helped me see and believe in the power of a woman's body. She was a huge influence on me and what I wanted for my future birthing experience. Sue was supposed to be my midwife, but very sadly she passed away from cancer in 2017.

When it was my turn to be a mama, I asked my husband, Thinus, if we could attempt a home birth. At first, he was not on board. However, our future midwives assured us that if we chose to birth at home they would transfer us to the hospital before any potential risk could become an emergency. He finally agreed when I suggested that we ask my good friend Pearl and her mom Judy if we could use their spacious home (and beautiful garden) instead of our apartment, which was too close to neighbors for comfort. They kindly agreed, and we began the preparations.

I thoroughly enjoyed this process of getting all the logistics of birth in place. I had lists of things to get prepared, like my labor bag with comfy clothes, pajamas, and maternity pads. And then the home birth list of old towels, bed linen, plastic coverings for the mattress and the floor, big buckets for the soiled linen after the birth, a container for the placenta, a birth ball, fairy lights to hang, and menus to plan for me and my team! As environmentally unfriendly as straws are, we were advised to get "bendy" straws so that no matter what position I was in, I could drink fluids. The straws did come in most handy! I also made sure all the administration was done with the medical aid, found out what emergency service was nearby, and saved their number to be prepared. Being a midwife, I knew this was wise and safe. We prepared the space little by little in the weeks before my due date. By the time I went into labor, the mattress was covered in plastic under the old linen, and the room was draped with fairy lights! It was all as I envisioned.

We invited our very close friends Jonathan and Jessie to be at the birth, as they are familiar with what is needed for a home birth and could support my husband, Thinus. Jessie would be my photographer, as I felt comfortable with her in my space. I also asked my mom to be part of the birth support team, and she was excited to accept the role!

I chose to birth with Birth Options, a practice with four very experienced midwives, and I had a wonderful obstetrician, Dr. Jacky Searle, as my backup. I chose Lana Peterson as my doula. I met Lana at Sue King's memorial service on Muizenburg beach. We didn't even speak that day, but her strength and gentle way of being really made an impression on me. When I needed a doula, I knew it had to be her. I didn't know her name, so I searched and found her on the Western Cape, South Africa doula list. I reached out to her, she remembered me from the beach memorial, and she accepted me as her client. What a wonderful road she walked with us.

I waited patiently for my little girl Maria Joy's arrival. I had a couple of interesting "letting go" experiences during my pregnancy. I was admitted into hospital twice, once at twenty-six weeks for bleeding (it didn't end up being serious) and again at thirty-six weeks for what they thought was preeclampsia developing. Thankfully, all these admissions opened my heart to Maria being born when and how she needed to be. This was important to establish as I had definite ideas of how I wanted everything to happen. I had to realize that this was her birth, not mine, and that no matter how or where it happened, it was her story.

In retrospect, I realize that I intuitively knew I wouldn't birth at home. When I met Dr. Jacky Searle at six weeks pregnant, I walked away from her gregarious, genuine consultation with a knowing that this amazing lady would be at the birth of my baby. Having an obstetrician at your birth means you are definitely not at home, but this knowing didn't stop me from planning a home birth, and she didn't stop me from aiming for a home birth even after my preeclamptic symptoms at thirty-six weeks and my advanced age (thirty-eight) labeled my pregnancy as risky. In the private sector in South Africa, this is unheard of, but she discharged me back to the midwives. What a special lady for giving me a chance to believe in myself and my baby.

I finally went into labor at forty-four weeks. We went over to Pearl's house at about 10 p.m. I had the TENs machine on and labored through the night, coping well. Lana arrived after she had dropped her girls at school, and Glynnis was at our home by mid-morning. My birth support team was all there and working on a puzzle! The atmosphere was as I wanted it: calm, normal, and lots of care, love, and support for all. When Glynnis checked me I was fully dilated, but Maria, although engaged, was still high up in my pelvis. My waters broke, and although they were stained with old meconium, her heartbeat was strong and consistent, regular and healthy. Thinus was excited because he expected her to be born soon. As a midwife, however, I managed my expectations, because I knew that "fully dilated" didn't necessarily mean imminent. How right I was!

I continued laboring, working with the surges, but Maria still wasn't descending so Glynnis asked me if I wanted to try actively pushing. I agreed. I love that she asked my permission. I felt so respected and valued. I had specified in my birth plan that as much as possible I wanted to experience the spontaneous fetal ejection reflex. But in my situation and due to Maria's journey through my pelvis, my labor was not progressing.

Glynnis included me in making decisions which empowered me to take responsibility for the outcome. I was not just a patient being managed. I was a woman being guided. I started pushing and continued pushing with the surges. It was a very powerful experience of strength, determination, perseverance, and focus. I had no sense of time. Thinus was amazing—he encouraged me constantly. He kept reminding me that I was doing this for our Maria Joy.

Glynnis and Lana were also exceptionally patient and encouraging. Glynnis was like my cheerleader, helping me to keep going. Maria's heartbeat kept strong, consistent, and healthy all the way. Although my cervix was fully dilated, the contractions were very far apart at seven to eight minutes, so I got to rest in between. Lana helped me change positions, massaged my back, gave me homeopathic remedies, held my hand, and encouraged me.

Glynnis, monitoring me closely, said that although we were making slow progress getting her down onto the perineum, the meconium was getting thicker, meaning my baby was starting to become distressed. She asked me if she could cut an episiotomy to help birth her sooner, as we both knew the risks of meconium aspiration into her lungs. I agreed. Again, I love that she included me in her decision-making.

We did everything we could. I tried my best to birth her, but I didn't manage to at home. Because we were prepared well by Lana, and had ensured we had the ambulance number saved, there was no stress when it came time to transfer to hospital. Everyone stayed calm and maintained the space. The ambulance was called, and things were prepared for us to transfer to hospital. It's strange, because I had very accurately envisioned how a transfer could happen, and in my mind's eye I needed my mom there. I was so grateful that she was able to come in, hug me, and just be there to pray.

The ambulance arrived about ten minutes after we called it in. I was able to walk to the ambulance, and in so doing, waved goodbye to my amazing birth support team who had finished two big puzzles during the day! Off we went on a very bumpy, fun, laughter-filled ride to the hospital. The two paramedics were really great. In between me pushing, we were deciding what code my case was; I got an orange code, with sirens through the traffic lights! I was not afraid. Glynnis was with me, and I trusted her judgment. We listened to Maria Joy's heartbeat, and she was amazingly strong. Hearing that "thud-thud" was motivating and encouraging.

We got to the hospital quickly and went straight to the labor ward where Jacky, my obstetrician, and Bernice, another midwife in the Birth Options team, were waiting. Jacky examined me, and Maria Joy had gone right up high again (I think it was the bumpy ambulance ride). Jacky said, "We are going to surgery." Glynnis protested and told her that we had managed to get Maria into my perineum, so Jacky looked at me and said, "Christy, I'm giving you one push, and then we are going to surgery."

When the next contraction came, I summoned all my strength and determination and pushed my hardest. I brought my baby back down onto my perineum. Jacky saw how well we had done and called for a kiwi (vacuum). Maria Joy was finally born crying her lungs out! What a relief. She was so strong and so well! She had been in a backward position, gazing at the stars; the most difficult position to be born in. I'm so grateful we had the team we did, otherwise I would have had to go to surgery. A lovely pediatrician came to check her, and he didn't even remove my baby from my chest. He listened to her heart and lungs, and all was well!

While Jacky stitched me up, Lana weighed Maria after the birth team tried guessing her weight: Nine pounds! Twenty-two inches! No wonder I had to work so hard and long to maneuver such a big, healthy baby through my pelvis. Lana then placed her on my chest to initiate breastfeeding. She latched and suckled like a pro.

After everything had calmed down and I was sorted out, we were moved to the ward where Maria Joy got skin-to-skin time with her Papa! Her granny was also there with us to welcome her. Once we were settled, Thinus and my mom had to go home. Thinus was absolutely exhausted and needed a good sleep after pouring out his care and support on us.

Maria Joy and I stayed together, skin-to-skin, in hospital the whole night. We were able to get the best start to our breastfeeding journey. Even though we weren't in our home setting, we were safe and cared for. All was well. I was so grateful. Even though I didn't get the birth I planned, I knew I had tried my absolute best. I was at peace.

Birth Options has a team of four midwives who take turns to see you through your pregnancy. They work on a call system, and it turned out that Glynnis was the midwife sent to be my guide and guardian that day. I did not foresee what kind of midwife I would need, but Sue King (my angel in heaven) took care of that. I needed a midwife who would shout out her encouragement, who would question me when I questioned her: "What must I do now, Glynnis?" "What does your body say, Christy-Joy?" I needed a midwife who could see that I had what it took to persevere. I needed a midwife who had a sense of humor, but who could call out the hard truth. I needed a midwife who could make a call about what I wanted and what I needed. I needed a midwife who could balance giving her all to give me what I wanted, but who listened to my baby and my body over the noise of recommendations. I needed a midwife who would war with me to push a big, stargazing posterior baby through my pelvis, to the point where she was close enough to be helped out without aspirating on the meconium she was passing. I needed a midwife who would be in this battle of second stage labor for a time longer than we expected, and to see me through to the birth of my baby. I got my heart's desire which was to hold my baby immediately after birth, latch my baby, and keep my baby skin-to-skin for the next twelve hours, breastfeeding on demand. I needed this midwife to empower me.

I need to acknowledge my incredible husband, who witnessed this difficult birth, who had to wait out the long intervals between contractions, who had to bear with me seeking the right position that would help our baby girl rotate, who had to hear me release the cries of earnest effort, who had to trust my choice of providers and respect my space. He had to see the reality of feminine power in all its messy, gory glory. I couldn't have done it without him. I underestimated how much I would need him. His encouragement and presence kept me focused and believing, pushing past myself to see our baby girl. His encouragement was different to that of Glynnis. Her encouragement spoke to my body while Thinus's encouragement spoke to my heart. I needed both to achieve the birth I wanted.

I feel honored and privileged to have made it through the veil to the other side—where you are no longer one being, but two. Where a part of yourself is outside of yourself. It is mind-blowing. It is raw, scary, messy, unexpected, dangerous, and powerful. I am now a mother. Exhale. I am an empowered mother, knowing that I am stronger than I ever knew.

Maalikah's Positive Birth Mindset

"I want women to know that being transferred from home to hospital does not mean that you lose all control of your birth experience. Staying positive and remembering that you are being cared for by professionals who are there for you and your baby's best interests are important as you want your new birth team to work with you, not against you. But also remember that you are in total control of your body, no matter where you birth."

—Maalikah, teacher
South Africa

After having forced Cesarean sections with my first two children at private hospitals, I was determined to have a natural birth with our third baby. I started phoning around at hospitals, but almost none wanted to assist as they categorized me as high-risk for a vaginal birth. I did find two hospitals that were prepared to help me, but birthing with them was going to be very expensive.

Ultimately, I decided to make an appointment at a public hospital where I got quite a lot of positive feedback. I also started researching home birth. I began calling a few midwives, but very few were prepared to accommodate me as I was categorized as high-risk due to the previous two Cesareans. I received a referral to a midwife, Ruth. I called her, made an appointment, and latched on to her right away. Ruth has a warm welcome, years of professional experience, a calm approach, and a positive mindset. Ruth gave me so much hope that I knew I was going to have a natural birth. I attended a few of her preparation workshops, and through one of these workshops I reunited with an old friend who also had two Cesareans, and with Ruth's assistance she had a natural birth with her third child. This gave me loads of confidence in Ruth and myself.

On November 20th, 2019 at 2:00 a.m. I started having intermittent pains. By 4:00 a.m. the pains were getting more frequent. I called Ruth and she came over with her assistant and confirmed that I was in labor. My husband took our kids to a family member's home while the midwives took care of everything and ensured I was comfortable at all times. They made the birthing room cozy and comfortable by lighting some good smelling aroma and dimming the lights. They did regular checks on baby's heartbeat. My husband was very supportive and rubbed my back to ease the pains. He played my favorite Koran recitation which helped keep me calm and kept my mind strong and occupied.

From 12:00 p.m. the pain became extremely strong. By now I've been pacing and panting up and down, feeling like I was going to faint. I don't know how I had been moving around the house. By 2:00 p.m., as I got up from bed, my water broke. Shortly after my water broke, I was fully dilated. Ruth told me it was time to push, and the midwives took turns assisting me with my husband by my side. They did regular checks and could feel the baby's head. I tried laying down and pushing. I tried a squatting position, leaned against the wall, then went into the shower. I sat on the toilet. By 5:00 p.m. I was extremely exhausted and just wanted the baby to come out.

By 6:00 p.m. the midwives consulted with me. Despite our best efforts, our baby wasn't making progress toward being born. Our baby's heartbeat was still normal, but delaying things longer could cause baby to go into distress or could cause some serious harm to me. I agreed that we should go to the hospital as I was fully dilated and the hospital would give me a chance to try birthing vaginally.

My husband helped me get into our car, and I laid on the backseat for the ten-minute ride to the maternity hospital. As we stopped at the entrance, the security officer got us a wheelchair and helped me out of the car and into one of the hospital rooms. The gynecologist and nurses did some checks. The gynecologist advised me that since I was a high-risk patient, it would be safer to do a Cesarean. My head started to pound and my heart started to race, as this is what I was fearing. But then the nurses told her that I was fully dilated, and they could feel the baby's head so we should give a vaginal birth a try. I felt a sense of relief as I had come this far with my natural birth. Everyone agreed, and they moved me to the labor ward.

The nurses guided me through pushing, and I pushed as hard as I could. Part of baby's head came out then, but went back in again. I pushed again. Again, our baby's head came out and went back in. This happened a few times and that's when they discovered baby was in posterior position. Then it all made sense to me why I was struggling to push baby out.

They then did a small incision, and encouraged me to push again. At this time, I felt completely exhausted and drained, but I remained positive and built up some strength to start pushing again. With each push our baby came further and further out.

My husband held my hand and encouraged me to push. About five nurses and the gynecologist were also standing around the bed encouraging me to push and telling me I could do it. I closed my eyes and said a prayer to myself knowing if this baby didn't come out now, I might end up with another Cesarean. I took a deep breath, used all my energy, and I pushed and pushed. Our baby was born at 9:50 p.m. on November 20th, 2019. What a blessing and relief when I held my precious baby girl. There were tears of joy and congratulations from the nurses on my new baby girl. The nurses and gynecologist were all amazed as it's very rare that they witness a vaginal birth after two Cesareans. A special thanks to Ruth, my husband and nurses. I could not have done it without their support.

A Peaceful Transfer
in South Africa

○ ○ ○ ○ ○ ○ ○ ○ ○ ○ ○ ○ ○ ○ ○ ○ ○ ○

"Birth is a sacred journey for both mother and child. Some people may fear birth as it's a journey into the unknown—no two births are the same—however, if you remember women have been doing this for centuries and find the right support structure for your birth experience, it can take place without fear present. Home birth gives you the best of both worlds: at-home care, comfort, safety, and privacy as well as on-call medical support when needed."

—Emma
Cape Town, South Africa

It was a Tuesday morning when my partner, Jason, asked several times if it would be okay for him to go to his meetings. I said, "of course" as I wasn't expecting anything to happen that day and knew he'd be there if I needed him back home. I knew the baby wouldn't come out in say, thirty minutes, so if something did happen, he would be there in time. Maybe he instinctively knew things were beginning to happen. I had increased surges coming more frequently over the last day or two, but one doesn't know for how long surges will continue until the real thing begins. I had a Skype conversation around 10:00 a.m. that morning with a dear friend, but found I couldn't concentrate well, and I kept it short. I think I went to bed to rest and Jason asked me to check in every hour.

Jason had conveniently downloaded a surge tracker on my phone so I could time each surge and send him updates. The surges started getting a little stronger, and I could see the shape of my belly changing each time it contracted. I sent Jason a photo. I got to a point where I found it difficult to focus and concentrate and told Jason he should come home. He must have contacted Marianne, our midwife, who then called me, but I found it hard to concentrate and talk so I couldn't answer her questions very well. She or Jason must have called Lana, our doula, and she arrived first. It was hard work to message, stand up, answer the phone to let her in at the gate, and unlock the door. But I pushed myself to do it and was thankful to go back to the bed.

It was a relief to have loving support from someone who was 100 percent there for me. I even cry now. Her gentle voice and touch were reassuring and comforting. It meant the world to me and helped me so much. I remember vomiting into a bag Lana found while Jason pulled my hair back and put it up. I felt most comfortable in bed, lying in a semi-reclined position.

Marianne arrived not long after Lana. She wore a beautiful blue top to mark the occasion. I felt honored she had "dressed up" for me. She, like so many independent midwives, is a gifted mother divine to many. I was grateful to have the love and support of these two beautiful women who nurtured and empowered me as needed. Jason arrived soon after. I learned that he had been out in Stellenbosch and traffic had been bad, so that's what had taken him a while to get here. He held my hand sometimes. I leaned on Lana's chest and held her hand, I held Marianne's hand, and the surges continued. Everyone took turns as the afternoon turned into evening. The intensity grew gently. There was some pain in my lower back with the surges as I was semi-reclined. It may not have been the best position while in a surge, but it was hard work to move, so I felt better to stay. This continued on during the night. I remember hearing someone snore as I dozed on and off. I don't remember many details of the night.

As morning came, the surges continued. Sometime that morning I had a shower. It was relaxing and provided some soothing pain relief being under the running water. Someone was always with me. I think Lana helped me into the shower then swapped with Marianne. They must have all been very tired. When asked if I wanted to get in the pool, I said, "yes!" It was a relief to be in the pool. I could feel the surges coming, but I didn't want him to come out yet. I asked him to take his time. Jason got in with me for a while, and it was nice to lean against him. He didn't stay in for long. He also sat outside the pool and read me birth affirmations. I appreciated that. So sweet and thoughtful, and it took my attention away from the intensity.

I hadn't eaten so they were giving me water and coconut water to sip through a straw. While in the pool we tried rice, but I just couldn't stomach it and didn't want it. I just couldn't eat it. I had felt just slightly nauseous through the labor and really didn't want to swallow or eat anything..

I'm not sure how long I was in the pool (thank you to those who set it up and filled it up). My surges started slowing down so the wonderful Marianne said it was time to get out. We needed to move the process along, so back to the bed we went. I then had to "roast the chicken" to help get the baby in a better position. This meant lying on one side for about ten minutes, then the other, and continue alternating for an hour or two. I didn't like lying on my side as it was more uncomfortable and intense during the surges, but in between contractions it was okay. They also said I needed to start pushing with each surge to help him move down. Marianne came in a bit later and asked me if I wanted to stop or go somewhere else. I said I didn't want to stop because I could feel progress picking up and could get the baby further down.

After some time, Marianne said we should go to the bathroom so off we went.

As the surges continued and baby came down, Lana stood behind me with her arms under my shoulders while she sat in front of me. After a few more surges our baby arrived!

Marianne wiped him a bit and noticed he was breathing very quickly. She suctioned him by sticking a clear pipe down his mouth and sucking out liquid (he was frothing a little at the mouth), then down the nose. She checked him quickly and did it again. Then I held him in my arms. They helped me back to the bed and baby came with me. They put him on oxygen by putting pipes up his nose. He was born at 8:40 p.m. on Wednesday.

Lana said we should have taken a photo of her face when the baby came out—he was massive at ten pounds! Lana also said the placenta was very large. While he was still on oxygen, our baby looked to have respiratory distress (breathing faster than he should be). Marianne said we should take him to hospital. There was a chance there was meconium in the waters and he swallowed some. She started calling the closest public hospital, but she wasn't getting anywhere. Jason suggested we go to a private hospital as we had insurance, so Marianne phoned them and said a pediatrician would be there waiting for us. I knew Marianne and Lana were doing the right thing, and this is what our baby needed. I was calm and grateful to have this firsthand support. I was not worried or distressed.

Jason had our baby on his chest while they helped me wash and get dressed. Jason went down to the car with our baby. Marianne and Lana helped me to the car. While we drove, Marianne and Lana stayed at the house and cleaned up. They even made our bed with fresh sheets. Marianne would join us at the hospital soon after. Such incredible, steadfast commitment and support.

A nurse and a doctor from the Neonatal Intensive Care Unit was waiting for us at the door. They took our baby and explained what they were going to do. We stayed for a little while then went home. I knew he was in good hands. The transition and support of the midwife and doula was beyond expectations. They are so experienced in what they do.

We visited him each day and could hold him. They allowed me to breastfeed with him which was so wonderful. I'll never forget the first time he latched. Dear Marianne and Lana visited us at the hospital as well. This extra care was so kind and thoughtful of them. I knew our baby was in good hands, and he had to be there. I knew our energy and attitude were important, and we could talk about it with our precious baby as well. Looking back, he was in hospital for only four nights, and I was able to stay with him on the last night.

When we arrived on Saturday morning the doctor on duty looked very serious. I thought she would definitely be keeping him in. To my utmost surprise, her first words were about getting him home. She wanted everything taken off (drip, oxygen) and just another blood test done to check for jaundice. I was so happy she was so supportive of getting him home!

They arranged for me to stay in one of the beds that night to check that his breathing was okay before releasing him. We had a little monitor we had to keep attached which monitored his heartbeat. We had a lovely nurse, Crista, who would come in and check on us and help with feeding if he wasn't latching well. He was all checked out by the doctor by 8:30 a.m. the next morning. Jason arrived Sunday morning, and we had to fill out a few forms, and the lovely head nurse was so kind and helpful. Then it was into the car and home! Our baby slept all the way home.

Words of thanks cannot even partly express my gratitude for my midwife and doula. They will forever be dear friends and fellow sisters for life. I may be but a drop in the ocean to them, but to me, they mean the world and fill my heart with continuous love and joy. They will never be forgotten. They held me, supported me, tenderly cared for me, and held my hand as I entered the world of motherhood.

Acknowledgments

○ ○ ○ ○ ○ ○ ○ ○ ○ ○ ○ ○ ○ ○ ○ ○ ○ ○ ○

This book was a sliver of a dream. It was made a reality by the support of the twenty-nine contributors, their midwives, photographers, doulas, and partners. The time and energy spent contributing to this collection of stories was substantial. I am forever grateful for the openness and honesty written within these beautiful home birth stories.

○ ○ ○ ○ ○ ○ ○ ○ ○ ○ ○ ○ ○ ○ ○ ○ ○ ○ ○

I would also like to thank Jois and Marla for their wisdom, friendship, and enthusiastic support, my mom for everything, my husband for being a true partner and supporter of my dreams, and my midwives, Mary and Pita, for showing me the beauty of midwifery and motherhood.

○ ○ ○ ○ ○ ○ ○ ○ ○ ○ ○ ○ ○ ○ ○ ○ ○ ○ ○

Skyhorse Publishing and my editor, Nicole Mele, have been an amazing team to work with. I'm so pleased they said "yes!"